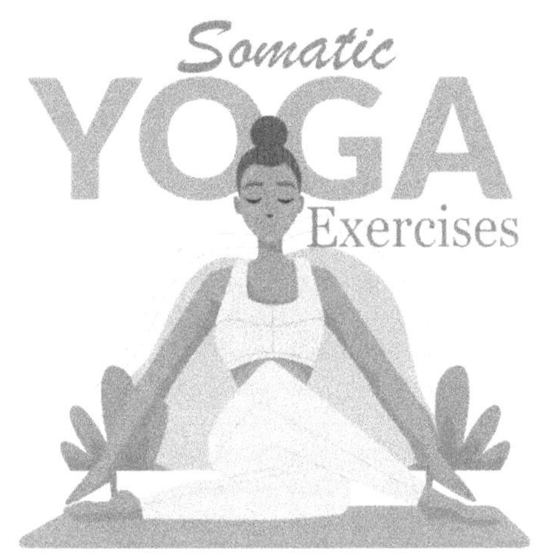

Somatic
Yoga Exercises
for Weight Loss

A Holistic 30-Day Somatic Yoga Plan for Stress Reduction, Weight Loss, Emotion Balancing, Pain Management, and Restorative Poses for Achieving Flexibility and Mobility

By

Michelle W. Vogel

Copyright

Disclaimer

The exercises and advice contained within this book, "Somatic Yoga Exercises for Weight Loss," are intended for informational purposes only. They are not a substitute for professional medical advice, diagnosis, or treatment. The author, Michelle W. Vogel, and the publishers do not assume any liability for injuries or health conditions that may result from following the exercise routines presented herein.

Before beginning any new exercise program, including the somatic yoga exercises detailed in this book, it is recommended that you consult with your physician or healthcare provider. Individual weight loss results may vary, and the effectiveness of the exercises may differ based on individual fitness levels, body types, and commitment to the program.

The author and publishers have made every effort to ensure the accuracy and efficacy of the exercises and information presented, but they cannot guarantee that the techniques will be suitable for every individual reader. Readers are encouraged to approach the exercises with mindfulness and to adapt them to their personal capabilities and needs.

By using this book, you acknowledge and agree that you are doing so at your own risk, and you willingly accept responsibility for any potential adverse effects on your health.

Introduction

In the quiet early hours of a spring morning, I found myself standing in front of a full-length mirror, scrutinizing every curve and contour of my body. For years, I had battled with weight gain, trying countless diets and grueling workout regimens. Yet, the results were often temporary, and the journey was fraught with frustration and disappointment. It wasn't until I stumbled upon somatic yoga that everything began to change. This book, "Somatic Yoga Exercises for Weight Loss," is a culmination of that transformative journey, and it is my heartfelt hope that it will serve as a beacon of inspiration and guidance for you, just as it did for me.

The Journey Begins

Our journey begins not with a grueling workout or a strict diet, but with a story—my story. A story that, perhaps, mirrors your own in many ways. I was an ordinary person, caught in the relentless cycle of weight gain and loss, feeling defeated and exhausted by the myriad of solutions that promised quick fixes but delivered little lasting change. One day, a friend suggested I try somatic yoga. Skeptical but desperate, I agreed.

As I lay on my mat, focusing on gentle, mindful movements and deep, restorative breaths, I began to feel a shift—not just in my body, but in my mind and spirit. This wasn't just about burning calories or shedding pounds; it was about reconnecting with my body, understanding its needs, and nurturing it with compassion and care. Somatic yoga became a sanctuary, a space where I could heal and grow, both physically and emotionally.

You see; "Somatic Yoga Exercises for Weight Loss" is not just a book; it's a journey into the depths of self-discovery and healing. Authored by the compassionate and insightful Michelle W. Vogel, this guide is a beacon of hope for those who have wandered through the maze of weight loss solutions, only to find themselves at the starting point again. Michelle's approach is different; it's holistic, gentle, and grounded in the wisdom of somatic practices that reconnect you with the innate intelligence of your body.

As you turn these pages, you will embark on a path that transcends the traditional narrative of weight loss. This book is a tapestry woven with the threads of mindfulness, movement, and breath, inviting you to explore the somatic exercises that will transform your physique but as well as nourish your soul. Each chapter is a stepping stone towards a lighter, more vibrant version of yourself, where the goal is to shed pounds and shed the layers of self-doubt and limitation.

Michelle W. Vogel's voice is a gentle whisper in your ear, encouraging you to move, to breathe, to feel. Her words are a soothing balm, healing the wounds inflicted by years of negative self-talk and unrealistic beauty standards. Through her guidance, you will learn to listen to your body's subtle cues, to honor its needs, and to celebrate its strength and resilience. The somatic yoga exercises presented here are more than physical postures; they are keys to unlocking the joy of living in a body that feels like home.

This book is a treasure chest of knowledge, brimming with detailed instructions, personal anecdotes, and the science behind somatic practices. Michelle's expertise as a seasoned yoga instructor and her personal experiences with weight loss infuse each page with authenticity and wisdom. She doesn't just teach; she walks alongside you, sharing her own vulnerabilities and victories, making the journey deeply personal and relatable.

As you delve deeper into "Somatic Yoga Exercises for Weight Loss," you will find yourself in the company of a community of readers who, are seeking a more meaningful connection with their bodies. You will learn that weight loss is not a race but a rhythm, one that ebbs and flows with the melody of your life's unique circumstances. This book is an invitation to dance to that rhythm, to embrace the fluctuations, and to find balance in movement and stillness.

Michelle's narrative is a mosaic of inspiring stories, practical advice, and heartfelt encouragement. She reminds us that everybody is a work of art, deserving of care and reverence. The somatic yoga exercises are her brushstrokes, painting a picture of health and harmony that is attainable for everyone, regardless of age, size, or fitness level.

In this introduction, we have only skimmed the surface of the rich content that awaits you. "Somatic Yoga Exercises for Weight Loss" is a guide, a friend, and a testament to the enduring spirit of those who choose to embark on this transformative journey. It is a book that will be revisited time and again, each reading offering new insights and deeper understanding.

So, take a deep breath, open your heart, and prepare to meet yourself on the mat with kindness and curiosity. Welcome to the world of Somatic Yoga, where every movement is an act of self-love, and every breath is a step towards a lighter, freer you.

How To Use This Book

This book is divided into several key sections, each serving a unique purpose in your journey:

Introduction to Somatic Yoga: Here, you'll learn about the fundamentals of somatic yoga, its principles, and how it differs from other yoga styles. This section provides a solid foundation to understand the techniques and practices that follow.

Getting Started: This section covers the basics of starting your somatic yoga practice, including choosing the right equipment, creating a comfortable practice space, and setting realistic goals. Foundational exercises are introduced to help you ease into your practice.

Daily Mindful Meditations: Incorporating mindfulness is crucial for achieving lasting weight loss. This section offers guided meditations to complement your physical practice, promoting mental clarity, relaxation, and a positive mindset.

Somatic Yoga Exercises: This is the core of the book, where you'll find detailed instructions for various somatic yoga exercises. Each exercise is designed with weight loss and body awareness in mind, providing step-by-step guidance, benefits, and modifications.

30-Day Somatic Yoga Routine: To help you integrate somatic yoga into your daily life, we've provided a 30-day workout plan. This structured plan ensures you have a balanced routine that targets different areas of the body, while also offering variety to keep you engaged.

30-Day Nutritional Plan: Complementing your yoga practice with proper nutrition is essential for weight loss. This section includes a detailed nutritional plan, complete with recipes and tips to support your goals.

Tracking Progress: Monitoring your progress is key to staying motivated and achieving your goals. This section offers tools and templates for tracking your practice, improvements in flexibility, strength, stress levels, and overall progress.

Yearly Progress and Conclusion: Reflect on your journey over the course of a year, setting new goals and celebrating your achievements. This section also offers advice on maintaining your practice and continuing your somatic yoga journey.

Approaching the Book

To get the most out of "Somatic Yoga Exercises for Weight Loss," follow these guidelines:

Read Thoroughly: Begin by reading through the introductory sections to understand the basics of somatic yoga and how it can benefit your weight loss journey. Familiarize yourself with the foundational exercises before moving on to the more advanced routines.

Start Slow: If you're new to yoga or physical exercise, start with the beginner-friendly exercises and gradually work your way up. Listen to your body and don't rush through the routines. Progress at a pace that feels comfortable for you.

Follow the 30-Day Routine: The 30-day somatic yoga routine is designed to give you a structured plan that builds strength, flexibility, and mindfulness. Stick to the plan as closely as possible, but feel free to make adjustments based on your personal needs and schedule.

Incorporate Mindfulness and Nutrition: Use the daily mindful meditations to enhance your mental well-being and support your physical practice. Follow the nutritional plan to ensure you're fueling your body with the right foods to support weight loss and overall health.

Track Your Progress: Use the tracking tools provided to monitor your practice and progress. Reflect on how your body and mind are responding to the exercises and make notes of any changes you observe. This will help you stay motivated and see the tangible benefits of your efforts.

Stay Consistent: Consistency is key to achieving lasting results. Aim to practice somatic yoga regularly, even if it's just for a few minutes each day. The cumulative effect of regular practice will lead to significant improvements over time.

Listen to Your Body: Always prioritize your body's needs and limitations. If you experience any discomfort or pain, modify the exercises or take a break as needed. Somatic yoga is about creating a harmonious connection between your mind and body, so always practice with compassion and mindfulness.

Create a Routine: Establish a routine that fits into your lifestyle. Whether you prefer practicing in the morning to energize your day or in the evening to unwind, find a time that works best for you and stick to it.

Join a Community: Consider joining a somatic yoga class or online community. Sharing your journey with others can provide support, motivation, and additional resources to enhance your practice.

Be Patient: Weight loss and physical transformation take time. Be patient with yourself and trust the process. Celebrate small victories along the way and remain committed to your goals.

Enjoy the Journey: Remember that somatic yoga is not just about weight loss; it's about nurturing a healthier, more mindful relationship with your body and mind. Enjoy the journey and embrace the positive changes that come with it.

Getting Started with Somatic Yoga

Choosing the Right Equipment

Embarking on your somatic yoga journey requires minimal equipment, making it accessible to everyone. We are going to look at all the equipment and essentials needed for our yoga journey.

Yoga Mat: A high-quality yoga mat provides a non-slip surface and cushioning for your joints. Look for a mat with adequate thickness (usually around 4-6mm) to ensure comfort during your practice.

Comfortable Clothing: Wear clothes that allow for a full range of motion. Choose breathable, stretchy fabrics that won't restrict your movements. Avoid overly loose clothing that might get in the way during poses.

Props: While not strictly necessary, yoga props can enhance your practice. Consider having a few items on hand, such as:

Yoga Blocks: Useful for modifying poses and providing support.

Yoga Strap: Helps in deepening stretches and achieving proper alignment.

Bolster or Cushion: Offers additional support for seated and reclining poses.

Blanket: Can be used for added comfort and support in various poses.

Water Bottle: Staying hydrated is important during any physical activity, including yoga. Keep a water bottle nearby to ensure you're drinking enough water throughout your practice.

Creating a Comfortable Practice Space

Your practice space plays a crucial role in your somatic yoga experience. Let's look at some ways we can create an inviting and comfortable yoga environment:

Find a Quiet Spot: Choose a space where you can practice without distractions. This could be a dedicated room, a corner of a room, or even an outdoor area. The key is to find a place where you can focus and relax.

Ensure Ample Space: Make sure you have enough room to move freely. Clear away any clutter that might get in your way. Ideally, you should have enough space to fully extend your arms and legs in all directions.

Control the Lighting: Soft, natural light is ideal for yoga practice. If natural light isn't available, use soft, warm lighting. Avoid harsh, bright lights that can be distracting and create a sense of discomfort.

Set the Mood with Music: Gentle, calming music can enhance your yoga practice. Choose instrumental music or nature sounds that help you relax and focus. Create a playlist that you can play softly in the background.

Use Aromatherapy: Essential oils and incense can create a soothing atmosphere. Scents like lavender, eucalyptus, and sandalwood are particularly calming. Be mindful of any sensitivities or allergies you might have.

Setting Realistic Goals

Setting realistic goals is an essential part of your somatic yoga journey. Here's how to establish goals that are achievable and meaningful:

Start Small: If you're new to yoga or physical activity in general, start with short, manageable sessions. Aim for 10-15 minutes per day and gradually increase the duration as you become more comfortable.

Focus on Consistency: Consistency is more important than intensity. Commit to practicing regularly, even if it's just for a few minutes each day. Over time, this consistency will build a strong foundation for your practice.

Listen to Your Body: Pay attention to how your body feels during and after each session. Adjust your practice based on your energy levels, flexibility, and any discomfort you might experience. Avoid pushing yourself too hard, especially in the beginning.

Set Specific, Measurable Goals: Instead of vague goals like "get better at yoga," set specific, measurable goals. For example, you might aim to hold a particular pose for a certain amount of time or to practice a specific sequence without needing a break.

Celebrate Progress: Acknowledge and celebrate your progress, no matter how small. Keep a journal to track your achievements and reflect on how far you've come. Celebrating your successes will keep you motivated and engaged.

Foundational Exercises to Begin Your Journey

To help you get started, here are some simple, foundational exercises that introduce you to the principles of somatic yoga. These exercises focus on gentle movements, mindful breathing, and body awareness.

1. Somatic Breathing

Purpose: To connect with your breath and promote relaxation.

Instructions:

- Sit comfortably or lie down on your back.
- Place one hand on your abdomen and the other on your chest.
- Take a slow, deep breath in through your nose, allowing your abdomen to rise.
- Exhale slowly through your mouth, feeling your abdomen fall.
- Continue for 5-10 breaths, focusing on the sensation of your breath.

2. Pelvic Tilts

Purpose: To increase mobility in the lower back and pelvis.

Instructions:

- Lie on your back with your knees bent and feet flat on the floor, hip-width apart.
- Place your hands on your lower abdomen.
- Inhale and gently tilt your pelvis forward, arching your lower back slightly.
- Exhale and tilt your pelvis backward, pressing your lower back into the floor.
- Repeat for 10-15 repetitions, moving slowly and mindfully.

3. Cat-Cow Pose

Purpose: To improve spinal flexibility and relieve tension.

Instructions:

- Begin on your hands and knees, with your wrists under your shoulders and knees under your hips.
- Inhale, arch your back, and lift your head and tailbone towards the ceiling (Cow Pose).
- Exhale, round your spine, and tuck your chin and tailbone towards your chest (Cat Pose).
- Continue to alternate between Cat and Cow poses with each breath for 10-15 repetitions.

4. Somatic Arm Raises

Purpose: To promote shoulder mobility and coordination.

Instructions:

- Sit comfortably or stand with your feet hip-width apart.
- Inhale and slowly raise your right arm overhead, keeping your shoulder relaxed.
- Exhale and lower your arm back down to your side.
- Repeat with your left arm.
- Perform 10-15 repetitions on each side, focusing on smooth, controlled movements.

5. Seated Forward Fold

Purpose: To stretch the hamstrings and lower back.

Instructions:

- Sit on the floor with your legs extended straight in front of you.
- Inhale, lengthen your spine, and reach your arms overhead.
- Exhale, hinge at your hips, and fold forward, reaching towards your feet.
- Hold for 5-10 breaths, allowing your body to relax into the stretch.
- Slowly rise back up to a seated position.

By choosing the right equipment, creating a comfortable practice space, setting realistic goals, and beginning with simple, foundational exercises, you have laid the groundwork for a sustainable and fulfilling somatic yoga practice.

Remember, the key to success in somatic yoga is patience, consistency, and compassion for yourself. Embrace the journey, celebrate your progress, and enjoy the myriad benefits that somatic yoga brings to your body, mind, and spirit.

Understanding Somatic Yoga and Weight Loss

Understanding Somatic Yoga and Weight Loss involves recognizing how mindful movement, breathwork, and somatic awareness can enhance physical and mental well-being. By integrating these practices, you can improve body awareness, reduce stress, and support weight loss goals through mindful living.

What is Somatic Yoga

Somatic Yoga is a holistic approach to physical and mental well-being that integrates movement, breath, and awareness. It is a mindful movement practice that focuses on re-educating the mind-body connection to release tension, improve mobility, and restore natural movement patterns.

One of the key principles of Somatic Yoga is the concept of somatic awareness, which involves bringing conscious attention to the sensations and movements of the body. This awareness allows practitioners to identify areas of tension or restriction and work to release them through gentle, mindful movements.

Unlike traditional yoga, which often emphasizes static poses, Somatic Yoga involves slow, controlled movements that help to release chronic muscle tension and improve overall body awareness. By moving slowly and mindfully, practitioners can access deeper layers of tension and learn to release it, leading to greater ease and freedom of movement.

Somatic Yoga can be beneficial for people of all ages and fitness levels. It can help to improve flexibility, strength, and balance, as well as reduce pain and stiffness. It can also be a valuable tool for managing stress and anxiety, as the mindful movement and breathwork can help to calm the nervous system and promote relaxation.

Overall, Somatic Yoga is a gentle yet powerful practice that can help to improve both physical and mental well-being. By re-educating the mind-body connection and cultivating greater awareness, practitioners can experience greater freedom and ease in movement, as well as a greater sense of peace and calm in the mind.

The Science Behind Somatic Yoga

Somatic Yoga is more than just stretching and breathing; it's a method deeply rooted in the principles of somatic. This approach sees the body as a whole system, where every part is interconnected and affects the others. To understand how Somatic Yoga works, we dive into neuroscience, biomechanics, and psychology.

Our bodies develop movement patterns and habits over time, often leading to issues like muscle tension and limited mobility. Somatic Yoga aims to reprogram these patterns through gentle movements and focused attention. This process helps to release what's known as "sensory-motor amnesia," which is when your muscles stay contracted without you realizing it. By releasing this tension, your muscles can function better, giving you more flexibility and reducing pain.

The science behind Somatic Yoga is fascinating. As you practice, you're not just moving your body; you're also changing how your brain communicates with your muscles. This can have profound effects on your overall well-being, helping you move more freely and feel better both physically and mentally.

In essence, Somatic Yoga is a holistic approach that considers the entire body and mind, offering a path to greater living, health and vitality.

Benefits of Somatic Yoga for Weight Loss

As stated earlier, Somatic Yoga is a holistic practice that can benefit your weight loss journey in several ways. One of the key benefits of the Somatic Yoda Exercise is how it boosts body awareness and strengthens the connection between your mind and body. This heightened awareness can help you recognize and change unhealthy habits that might be hindering your weight loss efforts.

Another significant benefit of Somatic Yoga is its ability to reduce stress. Stress has been found to be a common factor in weight gain and can lead to emotional eating. By practicing Somatic Yoga Exercises regularly, you can learn to manage stress more effectively, reducing the urge to turn to food for comfort.

Also, Somatic Yoga Exercises can improve your overall sense of well-being. As you become more attuned to your body and its needs, you may find yourself naturally gravitating towards healthier foods and lifestyle choices. This, coupled with the stress-relieving effects of Somatic Yoga, can create a positive cycle that supports your weight loss goals.

Overall, Somatic Yoga Exercises is a gentle yet powerful practice that can complement your weight loss journey by promoting mindfulness, reducing stress, and improving your overall health and well-being.

How Somatic Yoga Differs from Traditional Yoga

Somatic Yoga and traditional yoga both aim to enhance the mind-body connection, but they do so in distinct ways. Traditional yoga typically involves holding poses to build strength and flexibility, whereas Somatic Yoga prioritizes gentle, flowing movements to alleviate tension and enhance mobility.

In Somatic Yoga, the focus is on internal awareness, prompting you to pay close attention to how your body feels during each movement. This level of awareness allows individuals to pinpoint areas of tension and release them, resulting in a more relaxed and supple body.

Another key difference lies in the approach to movement. Traditional yoga often follows predetermined sequences, while Somatic Yoga encourages practitioners to move in ways that feel natural and intuitive, allowing for greater freedom of expression.

Additionally, Somatic Yoga emphasizes the concept of pandiculation, which involves consciously contracting and then slowly releasing muscles to reset their resting length. This technique can help to reprogram the neuromuscular system, leading to improved muscle function and reduced pain.

Overall, while both forms of yoga offer numerous benefits for physical and mental well-being, Somatic Yoga's focus on gentle, mindful movements and internal awareness sets it apart as a unique and effective practice for enhancing the mind-body connection.

The Mind-Body Connection: How Somatic Yoga Aids in Weight Loss

The mind-body connection is a powerful force in our lives, especially when it comes to weight loss. Our thoughts, emotions, and habits can significantly impact our eating behaviors and physical activity levels. Somatic Yoga is a practice that focuses on strengthening this connection by emphasizing mindfulness and body awareness.

Through Somatic Yoga, you can develop a deeper understanding of your body's signals, such as hunger and fullness cues. This awareness can help you make more informed and mindful choices about your diet, leading to healthier eating habits and, ultimately, weight loss.

Furthermore, Somatic Yoga Exercise can also have a positive impact on body image. By practicing Somatic Yoga Exercise, you can develop a more positive relationship with your body, which can lead to a greater sense of self-acceptance and confidence. This, in turn, can motivate you to engage in regular physical activity and adopt a healthier lifestyle overall.

Somatic Yoga offers a holistic approach to weight loss by addressing both the physical and emotional aspects of wellness. By incorporating Somatic Yoga Exercise into your routine, you can nurture a deeper connection with your body, leading to lasting weight loss and improved overall health and well-being.

Breathing Techniques for Weight Loss

Breathing techniques are an essential aspect of any yoga practice, including Somatic Yoga, and can play a significant role in supporting weight loss efforts. In addition to providing the body with oxygen, proper breathing also lowers stress and enhances general wellbeing. In this section, we will explore several breathing techniques that can aid in weight loss.

1. Diaphragmatic Breathing

Also known as abdominal breathing, diaphragmatic breathing involves breathing deeply into the belly rather than the chest. This type of breathing can help to activate the parasympathetic nervous system, which promotes relaxation and reduces stress. Diaphragmatic breathing can also improve digestion and metabolism, which are important factors in weight loss.

To practice diaphragmatic breathing, sit or lie down in a comfortable position. Place one hand on your chest and the other on your abdomen. Take a deep breath in through your nose, allowing your abdomen to rise as you fill your lungs with air. Exhale slowly through your mouth, allowing your abdomen to fall. Repeat this process several times, focusing on the sensation of your breath moving in and out of your body.

2. Sitali Pranayama (Cooling Breath)

Sitali pranayama is a cooling breathing technique that can help to reduce body heat and calm the mind and nervous system. It involves inhaling through a rolled tongue (or pursed lips if you cannot roll your tongue) and exhaling through the nose. This breath is believed to have a cooling effect on the body and can help to reduce cravings and emotional eating.

To practice Sitali pranayama, sit in a comfortable position with your spine straight and shoulders relaxed. Roll your tongue into a "U" shape and inhale deeply through your mouth, allowing the breath to feel cool as it enters your body. Close your mouth and exhale slowly through your nose. Repeat this process for several breaths, focusing on the cooling sensation of the breath.

3. Kapalabhati Pranayama (Skull-Shining Breath)

Kapalabhati pranayama is a powerful breathing technique that can help to increase metabolism and promote weight loss. It involves rapid, forceful exhalations followed by passive inhalations. This breath is believed to cleanse the lungs and energize the body.

To practice Kapalabhati pranayama, sit in a comfortable position with your spine straight and shoulders relaxed. Take a deep breath in through your nose, then forcefully exhale through your nose, drawing your belly in towards your spine. Allow the inhalation to happen passively. Continue this rhythmic breathing for several rounds, gradually increasing the speed and intensity of the exhalations.

4. Nadi Shodhana Pranayama (Alternate Nostril Breathing)

Nadi Shodhana pranayama is a balancing breathing technique that can help to calm the mind and reduce stress. It involves alternating between breathing through the left and right nostrils, which is believed to balance the flow of energy in the body. This breath can help to improve digestion and metabolism, which are important for weight loss.

To practice Nadi Shodhana pranayama, sit in a comfortable position with your spine straight and shoulders relaxed. Use your right thumb to close your right nostril and inhale deeply through your left nostril. At the top of your inhale, use your right ring finger to close your left nostril and exhale through your right nostril. Inhale through your right nostril, then close it with your right thumb and exhale through your left nostril. Continue this pattern for several breaths, focusing on the smooth, even flow of your breath.

These breathing techniques can be practiced regularly to support your weight loss goals and enhance your overall well-being. Incorporating these techniques into your daily routine can help you to manage stress, improve digestion, and increase your metabolism, leading to more effective and sustainable weight loss results.

Somatic Yoga Poses for Core Strengthening and Toning

Core strength is essential for overall stability, posture, and movement efficiency. Somatic Yoga offers a unique approach to core strengthening by focusing on releasing tension and restoring natural movement patterns. The following poses can help you strengthen and tone your core muscles while promoting relaxation and body awareness.

1. Somatic Spinal Curl

Somatic Spinal Curl (SSC) is a movement in Somatic Yoga that focuses on releasing tension and increasing mobility in the spine. It is a full-body workout that targets the core and upper back muscles. It involves gently curling the spine forward, one vertebra at a time, and then slowly uncurling it back to a neutral position. This movement helps to improve flexibility and range of motion in the spine, while also promoting relaxation and body awareness.

How To Do This: Lie on your back with your knees bent and feet hip-width apart. Inhale to prepare, and as you exhale, gently tilt your pelvis and begin to lift your lower back off the mat, one vertebra at a time. Keep your core engaged, and your movements slow and controlled. Inhale at the top, then exhale to lower back down.

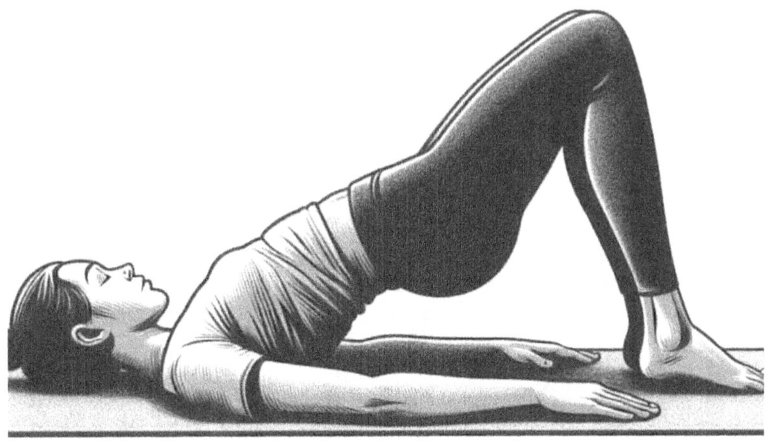

Duration: Hold each curl for a short time; 10–20 seconds, focusing on control and awareness rather than exertion.

Repetitions: 3–5 times for each side is a good starting point. Listen to your body and stop if you feel any pain.

Benefits: This pose strengthens the entire core, including the abdominal, obliques, and lower back. It also improves spinal mobility and flexibility.

2. Somatic Leg Lifts

Somatic Leg Lifts are gentle exercises in Somatic Yoga that target the muscles of the legs and lower body. They involve lifting one leg at a time while lying on your back, focusing on controlled movements and breath awareness. Somatic Leg Lifts help to improve leg strength, flexibility, and balance, while also promoting relaxation and mindfulness.

How To Do This: Lie on your back with your legs extended straight up towards the ceiling. Inhale to prepare, and as you exhale, engage your core and slowly lower one leg towards the floor. Keep your lower back pressed into the mat. Inhale to return to the starting position, then repeat on the other leg.

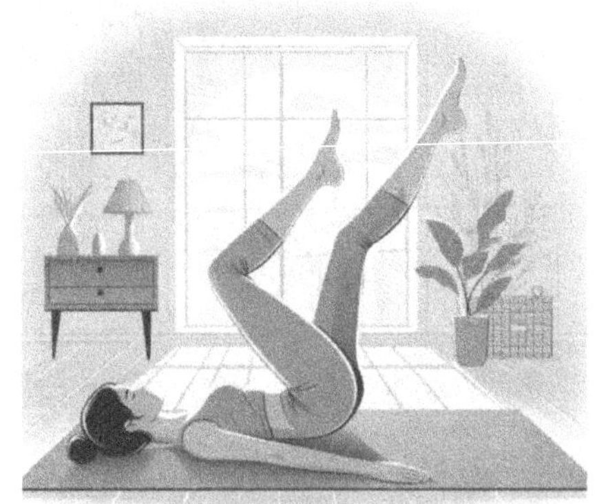

Repetitions: Begin with 5–10 movements per leg lift

Duration: Hold each lift for about 5–10 seconds, focusing on the sensation in your leg and how it connects to your body.

Benefits: This pose targets the lower abdominal and hip flexors, helping to tone and strengthen the core muscles.

3. Somatic Side Plank

Somatic Side Plank is a variation of the traditional side plank pose that is practiced in Somatic Yoga. In this variation, the practitioner lifts their body sideways, supporting themselves on one arm and the side of one foot, while lifting their hips to create a straight line from head to toe. Somatic Side Plank helps to strengthen the core muscles, improve balance, and increase overall body awareness.

How To Do This: Start in a plank position with your wrists under your shoulders and your body in a straight line from head to heels. Rotate onto the outer edge of your right foot and lift your left arm towards the ceiling, stacking your shoulders and hips. Hold for a few breaths, then return to plank and switch sides.

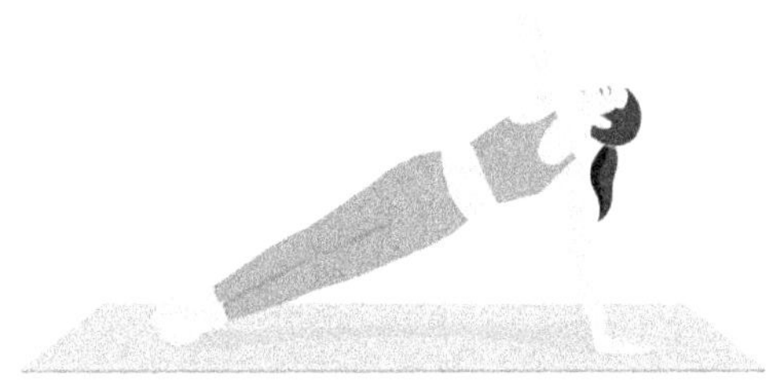

Duration: Start with holding the pose for about 15–30 seconds on each side

Repetitions: 3–5 repetitions per side

Benefits: This pose strengthens the obliques, shoulders, and arms while improving balance and stability.

4. The Boat Pose

The Boat Pose is a core-strengthening yoga pose that also engages the hip flexors and lower back muscles.

How To Do This: Sit on the floor with your knees bent and feet flat on the floor. Lean back slightly and lift your feet off the floor, balancing on your sit bones. Extend your arms straight out in front of you. Engage your core and straighten your legs if possible, forming a V shape with your body. Hold for a few breaths, then release.

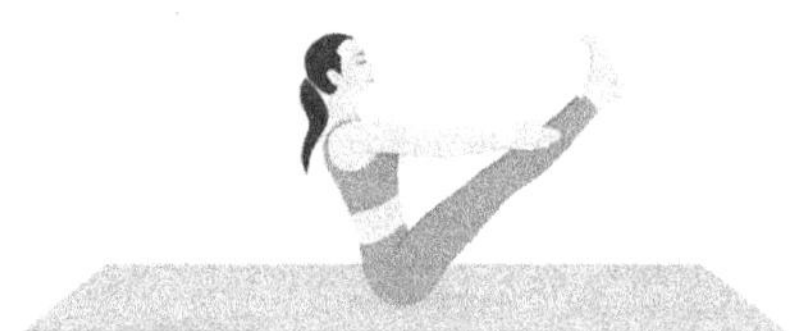

Duration: Hold each leg lift for a short time; 15–30 seconds.

Repetitions: 3–5 repetitions per leg is great for starters

Benefits: Boat pose strengthens the entire core, including the abdominal, obliques, and hip flexors, while also improving balance and posture.

5. Somatic Bridge Pose

Somatic Bridge Pose is a yoga pose that strengthens the core, glutes, and hamstrings while also improving spinal mobility. Bridge Pose helps to improve posture, alleviate back pain, and strengthen the lower body.

How To Do This: Lie on your back with your knees bent and feet hip-width apart. Press into your feet and lift your hips towards the ceiling, engaging your glutes and core. Hold the pose for a few breaths, then slowly lower your hips back down to the floor.

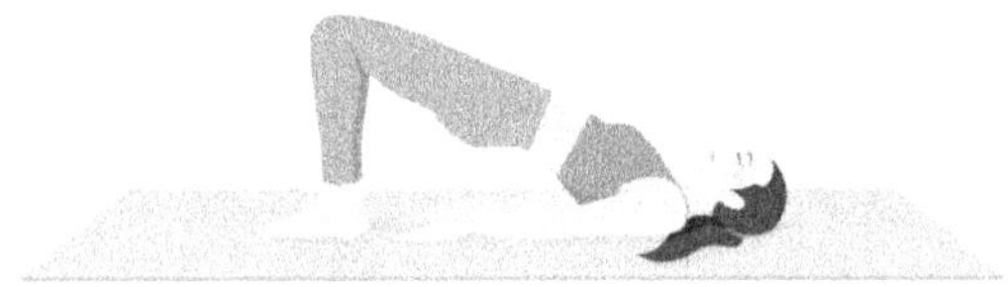

Duration: For starters, hold the pose for about 1–5 minutes.

Repetitions: 3–5 repetitions

Benefits: Bridge pose strengthens the core, glutes, and hamstrings, while also improving spinal mobility and posture.

6. Somatic Cat-Cow Stretch

Somatic Cat-Cow Stretch is a gentle yoga flow that helps to improve spinal flexibility and release tension in the back and neck. This stretch helps to improve spinal mobility, relieve back pain, and promote relaxation.

How To Do This: Start on your hands and knees in a tabletop position. Inhale as you arch your back and lowering your belly towards the floor and lifting your head and tailbone towards the ceiling (Cow Pose). Exhale as you round your spine and tuck your chin towards your chest (Cat Pose). Continue flowing between the two poses, moving with your breath.

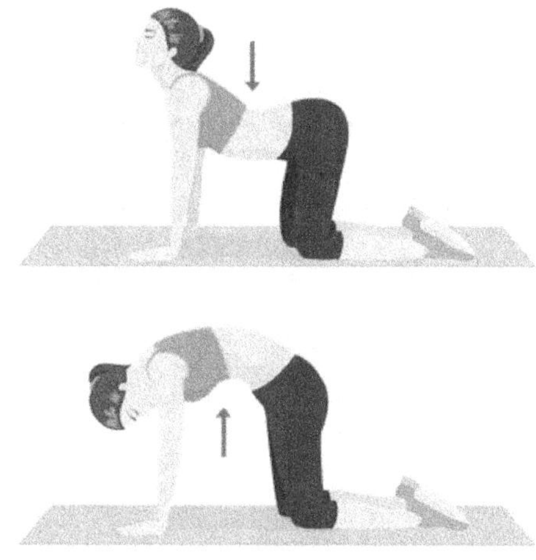

Duration: 1–2 minutes

Repetitions: Aim for 3–8 repetitions

Benefits: The Somatic Cat-Cow Stretch is great for improving spinal flexibility and mobility, while also strengthening the core muscles.

7. Somatic Plank Pose

Somatic Plank Pose is a core-strengthening yoga pose that also engages the arms, shoulders, and legs. This somatic yoga exercise helps to improve core strength, posture, and overall stability.

How To Do This: Begin in a push-up position with your hands directly under your shoulders and your body in a straight line from head to heels. Engage your core and hold this position for 30 seconds to 1 minute, or as long as you can maintain good form.

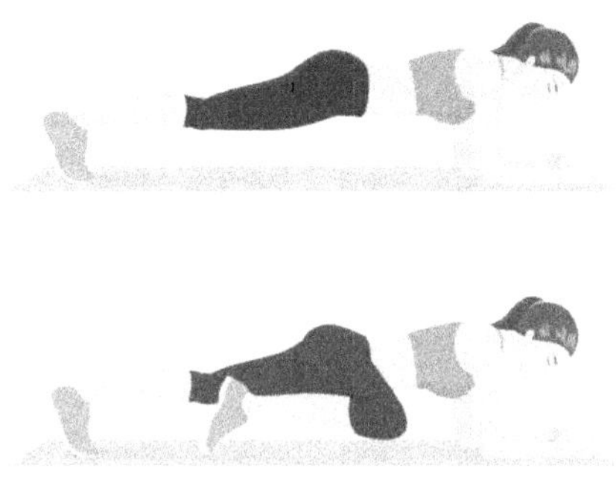

Duration: holding the pose for about 30– 60 seconds

Repetitions: Aim for 3–5 repetitions

Benefits: Plank pose strengthens the entire core, including the rectus abdominis, obliques, and transverse abdominis, as well as the shoulders, arms, and legs.

8. Somatic Knee-to-Elbow Plank

Somatic Knee-to-Elbow Plank is a variation of the traditional Plank Pose that targets the core muscles, particularly the obliques. This movement is aimed at strengthening the core, improving balance, and enhancing overall body awareness.

How To Do This: From plank pose, bring your right knee towards your right elbow, engaging your obliques. Hold for a moment, then return to plank and repeat on the left side. Continue alternating sides for several repetitions.

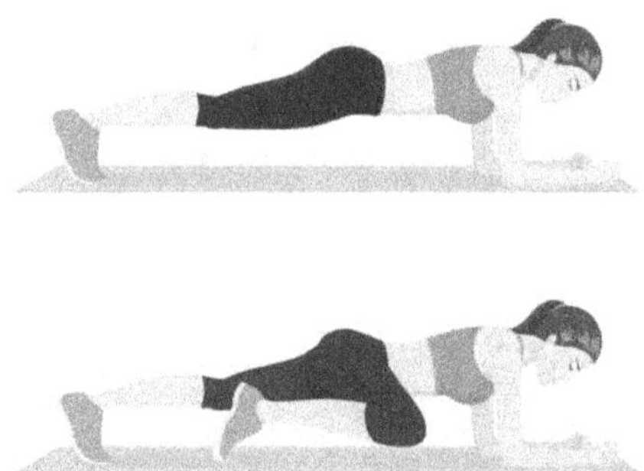

Duration: 10– 40 seconds

Repetitions: 5–10 repetitions on each side

Benefits: This variation of plank pose targets the obliques and hip flexors, helping to strengthen and tone the core muscles.

9. Pavanamuktasana or Somatic Wind-Relieving Pose

Somatic Wind-Relieving Pose, also known as Pavanamuktasana, is a yoga pose that helps to relieve gas and bloating in the abdomen. Wind-Relieving Pose helps to improve digestion, reduce bloating, and release tension in the lower back.

How To Do This: Lie on your back with your legs extended. Bring your right knee towards your chest, interlacing your fingers around your shin. Hold for a few breaths, then switch legs. You could also do this by bring both legs at the same time, gently hugging your knees towards your chest

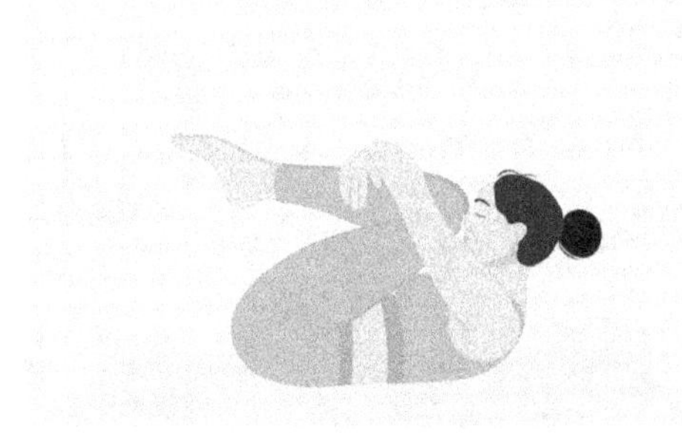

Duration: Hold the pose for about 20–30 seconds.

Repetitions: Aim for 3–5 repetitions, allowing yourself to relax and breathe deeply in the pose

Benefits: This pose helps to relieve gas and bloating in the abdomen, release tension in the lower back and hips, improves circulation, while also engaging the core muscles.

10. Somatic Seated Twist

Somatic Seated Twist is a yoga pose that helps to improve spinal mobility and release tension in the back. Seated Twist helps to stretch the spine, improve digestion, and relieve tension in the back and shoulders.

How To Do This: Sit on the floor with your legs extended straight out in front of you. Bend your right knee and place your right foot on the outside of your left knee. Inhale to lengthen your spine, then exhale to twist towards the right, placing your left elbow on the outside of your right knee. Hold for a few breaths, then switch sides.

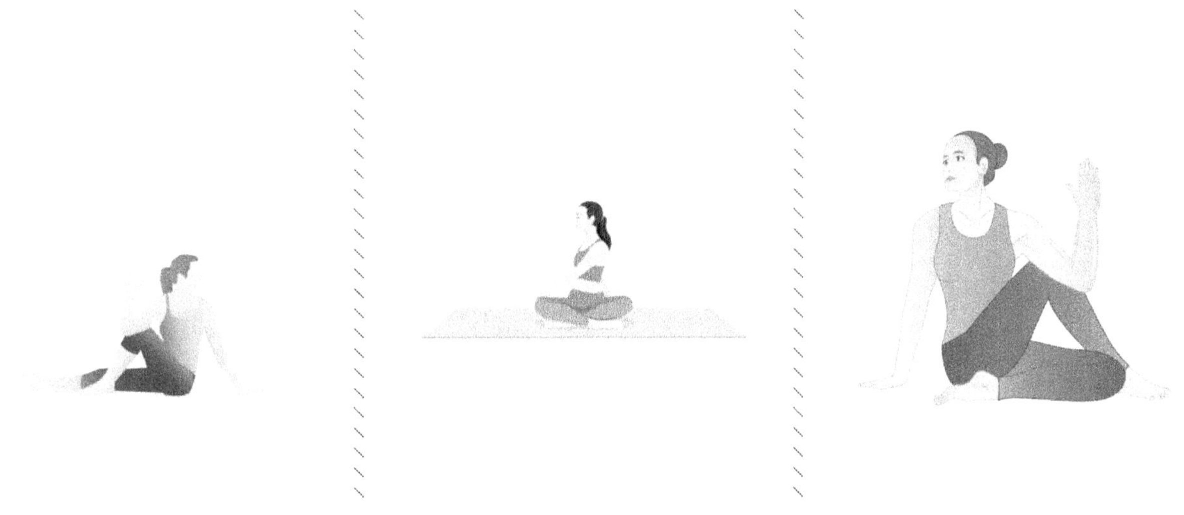

Duration: Hold the twist for about 20–30 seconds on each side.

Repetitions: Aim for 3–5 repetitions on each side.

Benefits: Seated twist pose helps to improve spinal mobility and digestion, while also toning the obliques and core muscles.

Practical Demonstration:

Before you carry out any of the somatic yoga exercises listed above, you need to be sure you are in a comfortable seated position, with your spine straight and shoulders relaxed.

Close your eyes and take a few deep breaths to center yourself.

Begin with the Somatic Spinal Curl, gently tilting your pelvis and lifting your lower back off the mat. And move towards the more advanced poses

Move through each pose slowly and mindfully, focusing on engaging your core muscles and maintaining proper alignment.

Remember to breathe deeply and stay relaxed throughout the practice.

End with a few moments of relaxation in Savasana, lying on your back with your eyes closed and your arms by your sides.

These Somatic Yoga poses can be practiced regularly to strengthen and tone your core muscles, improve your posture, and enhance your overall well-being.

Also listen to your body and modify or skip any poses that cause discomfort.

Somatic Yoga for Flexibility and Mobility

Flexibility and mobility are crucial for maintaining a healthy, active lifestyle. Somatic Yoga Exercises offers gentle yet effective poses to improve flexibility and mobility, focusing on releasing tension and increasing range of motion in the joints. These poses help to improve overall body awareness and reduce the risk of injury. Practicing these poses regularly can help enhance flexibility, improve posture, and increase mobility, leading to greater ease of movement and overall well-being.

1. Somatic Neck Release

Somatic Neck Release is a simple yet effective exercise to release tension in the neck and shoulders. This exercise helps to improve neck mobility, relieve neck pain, and reduce stiffness in the shoulders.

How To Do This: Sit or stand with your spine tall. Slowly tilt your head to one side, bringing your ear towards your shoulder. Hold for a few breaths, then return to center and repeat on the other side.

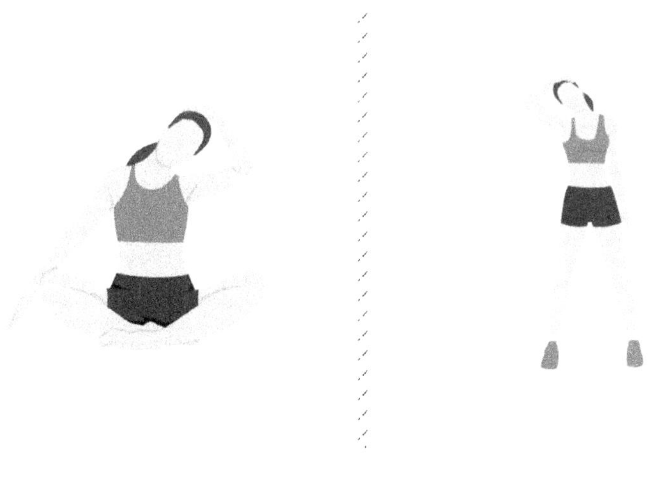

Repetitions: Repeat 4–8 times on each side.

Duration: Hold each stretch for 20–40 seconds.

Benefits: Relieves tension in the neck and shoulders, improves neck mobility.

2. Somatic Shoulder Stretch

Somatic Shoulder Stretch is a gentle exercise to release tension in the shoulders and upper back. This stretch helps to improve shoulder flexibility, reduce tightness, and promote relaxation in the upper body.

How To Do This: Reach one arm across your chest and use your other hand to gently press the arm towards your chest, feeling a stretch in the shoulder and upper back. Hold the stretch for a few seconds, then switch sides.

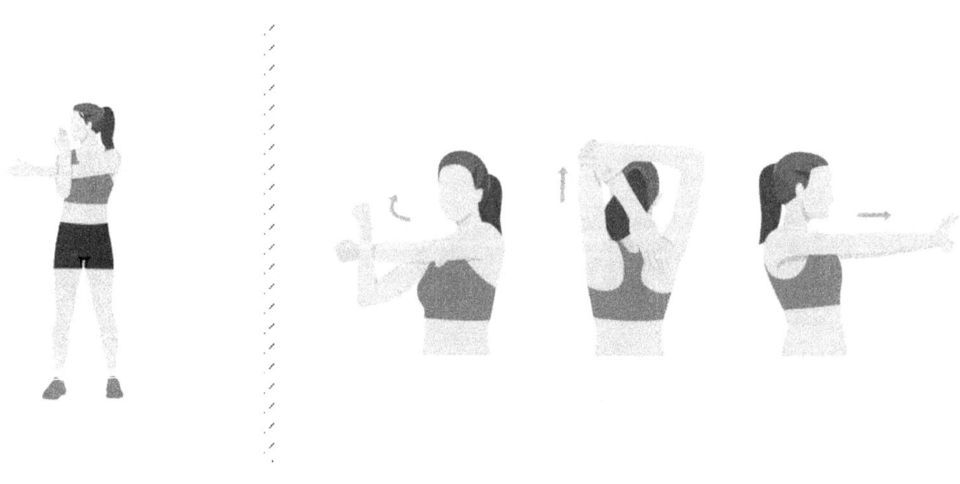

Repetitions: Repeat 3–5 times.

Duration: Hold for 20–30 seconds.

Benefits: Stretches the shoulders and chest, improves shoulder mobility.

3. Somatic Spinal Twist

Somatic Spinal Twist is a yoga pose that helps to improve spinal mobility and release tension in the back. This pose helps to stretch the spine, improve digestion, and relieve tension in the back and hips.

How To Do This: Lie down with your spine tall. Slowly twist your torso to one side, placing one hand on the opposite knee and the other hand on the floor behind you. Hold for a few breaths, then return to center and repeat on the other side.

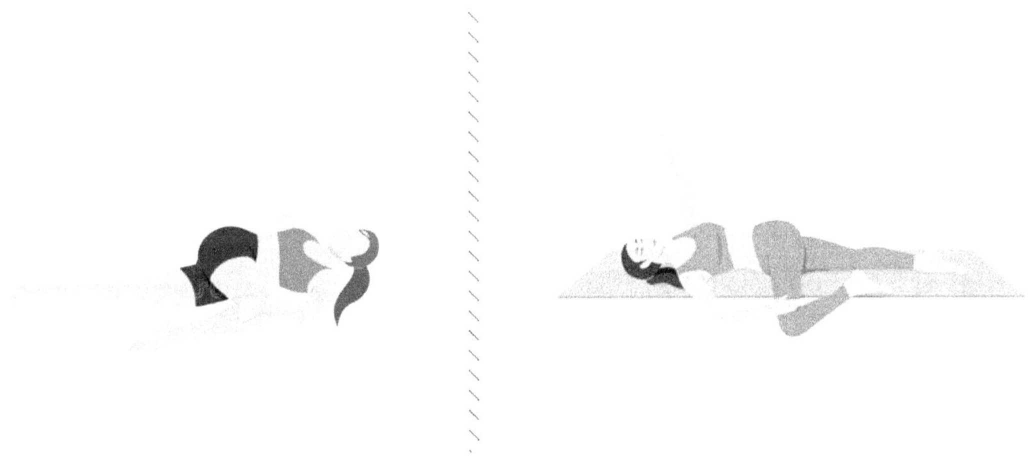

Repetitions: Repeat 3–5 times on each side.

Duration: Hold each twist for 15–30 seconds.

Benefits: Improves spinal mobility, stretches the back muscles.

4. Somatic Forward Fold

Somatic Forward Fold is a yoga pose that stretches the entire back body, including the spine, hamstrings, and calves. Forward Fold helps to release tension in the back, improve flexibility in the spine and hamstrings, and promote relaxation.

How To Do This: Stand with your feet hip-width apart and hinge forward at your hips, reaching towards the floor with your hands. Bend your knees slightly if needed. Relax your head and neck.

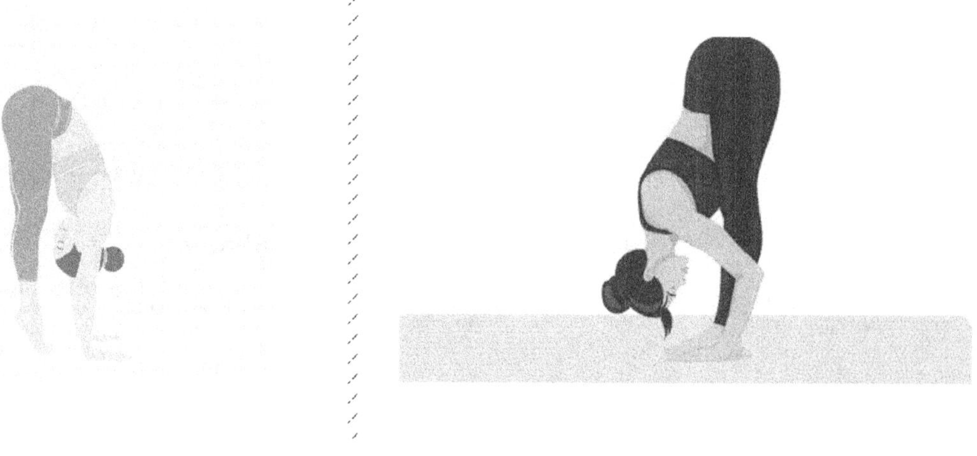

Repetitions: Repeat 4–8 times.

Duration: Hold for 20–30 seconds.

Benefits: Stretches the hamstrings and lower back, improves flexibility in the spine.

5. Somatic Hip Opener

Somatic Hip Opener is a yoga pose that helps to release tension in the hips and lower back. This pose helps to improve hip flexibility, reduce tightness in the hips, and alleviate lower back pain.

How To Do This: Sit on the floor with your legs extended in front of you. Bend one knee and place the sole of your foot on the opposite inner thigh. Lean forward slightly, keeping your spine tall.

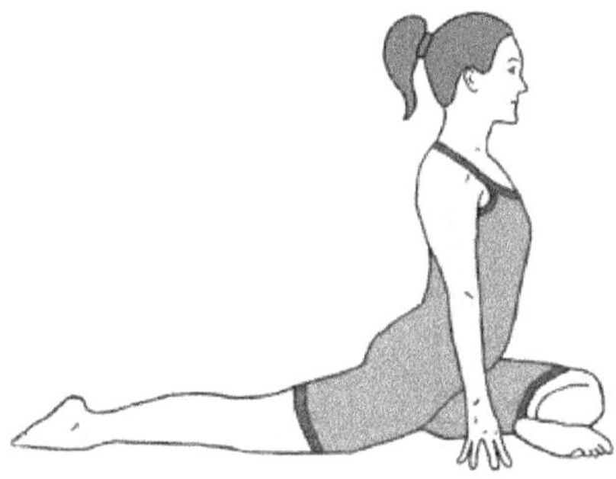

Repetitions: Repeat 3-5 times on each side.

Duration: Hold for 15-30 seconds.

Benefits: Stretches the hips and groin, improves hip mobility.

6. Somatic Butterfly Stretch

Somatic Butterfly Stretch is a yoga pose that helps to open up the hips and stretch the inner thighs. This pose helps to improve hip flexibility, reduce tightness in the inner thighs, and promote relaxation in the hips and lower back.

How To Do This: Sit on the floor with the soles of your feet together and your knees bent out to the sides. Hold onto your ankles and gently press your knees towards the floor. You can also lie on your back while performing the same stretch. Always make sure the sole of your feet are clapping each other.

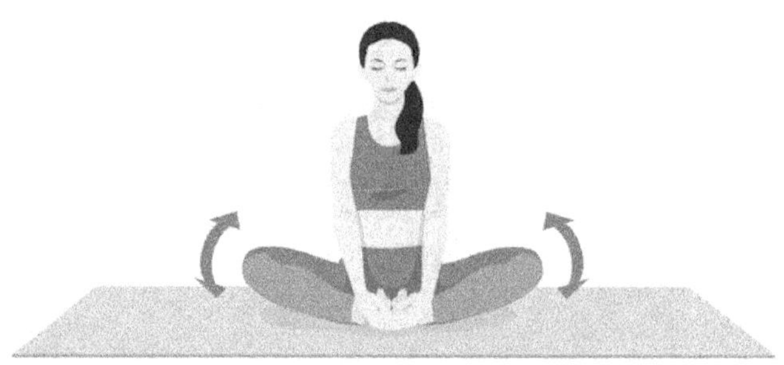

Repetitions: Repeat 4–8 times.

Duration: Hold for 20–40 seconds.

Benefits: Stretches the inner thighs and groin, improves hip mobility.

Practical Demonstration:

To do these poses, start by finding a quiet space where you can sit or stand comfortably. Focus on your breath and move slowly and mindfully through each pose, paying attention to how your body feels.

Remember to breathe deeply and relax as you perform each stretch to maximize the benefits.

Note: *It's important to listen to your body and modify the poses as needed to suit your level of flexibility and mobility. If you have any pre-existing injuries or conditions, consult with a healthcare professional before starting any new exercise program.*

Enhancing Metabolism through Somatic Yoga

Metabolism is the process by which your body converts the food you eat into energy. A healthy metabolism is crucial for maintaining a healthy weight and overall well-being. Somatic Yoga can help enhance metabolism by reducing stress, improving digestion, and increasing muscle mass. In this section, we will explore how Somatic Yoga can help enhance metabolism and improve overall health.

1. Stress Reduction

Stress can have a negative impact on metabolism by increasing the production of cortisol, a hormone that can lead to weight gain. Somatic Yoga helps reduce stress by promoting relaxation and mindfulness. By practicing Somatic Yoga regularly, you can lower your cortisol levels and improve your metabolism.

2. Improved Digestion

Digestion plays a key role in metabolism, as it determines how efficiently your body can extract nutrients from food. Somatic Yoga includes poses and breathing techniques that can help improve digestion by stimulating the digestive organs and promoting healthy digestion. Poses like gentle twists and forward bends can help massage the internal organs and improve digestion.

Somatic Yoga Exercise For Improved Digestion

Somatic Spinal Twist: This pose helps to stimulate digestion by massaging the abdominal organs and improving spinal mobility.

- **Somatic Wind-Relieving Pose (Pavanamuktasana):** This pose helps to release gas and bloating in the abdomen, aiding in digestion.

- **Somatic Seated Forward Fold:** This pose can help to stimulate digestion by compressing the abdomen and massaging the internal organs.

- **Somatic Child's Pose:** This resting pose can help to relax the abdominal muscles and aid in digestion.

- **Somatic Cat-Cow Stretch:** This gentle flow between cat and cow poses can help to improve spinal flexibility and stimulate digestion.

- **Somatic Downward-Facing Dog:** Improves digestion by lengthening the spine and promoting blood flow to the abdominal organs.

- **Somatic Bridge Pose:** Aids digestion by stretching the abdomen and stimulating the digestive organs.

- **Somatic Cobra Pose:** This gentle backbend can help to stimulate digestion by compressing the abdomen and massaging the internal organs.

3. Muscle Building and Toning

Muscle mass plays a crucial role in metabolism, because muscle burns more calories than fat. Somatic Yoga includes poses that can help build and tone muscles, especially in the core, legs, and arms. Poses like plank pose, boat pose, and lunges can help strengthen muscles and improve metabolism.

For more poses on muscle building and toning, refer to Somatic Yoga Poses For Core Strength and Toning

4. Increased Circulation

Somatic Yoga Exercises promotes increased blood flow and circulation, which can help improve metabolism. Better circulation means that nutrients and oxygen are delivered more efficiently to cells throughout the body, allowing them to function optimally. Poses that involve gentle inversions, like downward dog, Somatic Forward Fold (Uttanasana), Somatic Downward-Facing Dog, or legs up the wall pose, can help improve circulation and enhance metabolism.

5. Mindfulness and Eating Habits

Somatic Yoga encourages mindfulness, which can help improve eating habits and metabolism. By practicing mindfulness, you can become more aware of your body's hunger and fullness cues, leading to healthier eating patterns. Mindful eating can also help prevent overeating, which can negatively impact metabolism.

Practical Demonstration

To enhance metabolism through Somatic Yoga, incorporate the following practices into your routine:

Practice Somatic Yoga poses that focus on relaxation and stress reduction, such as child's pose, savasana (corpse pose), and gentle twists.

Include poses that stimulate digestion, such as seated forward bends, spinal twists, and gentle backbends.

Incorporate strength-building poses like plank pose, boat pose, and warrior poses to build muscle mass and increase metabolism.

Practice mindfulness both on and off the mat, paying attention to your body's hunger and fullness cues and making healthy food choices.

Combine Somatic Yoga with other forms of exercise, such as walking, jogging, or strength training, to further enhance metabolism.

Note: *It's important to listen to your body and practice Somatic Yoga mindfully. Consult with a healthcare professional before starting any new exercise program, especially if you have any pre-existing health conditions.*

Somatic Yoga for Stress Reduction and Weight Management

Stress is known to contribute significantly to weight gain and can make it challenging to manage weight effectively. Somatic Yoga presents a holistic approach to addressing stress, offering practices that not only reduce stress but also support weight management.

Somatic Yoga emphasizes gentle, flowing movements synchronized with deep breathing, promoting relaxation and reducing the production of stress hormones like cortisol. These practices can enhance mood, increase mindfulness, and improve overall well-being.

In this section, we will look at the specific Somatic Yoga poses and practices that can be particularly beneficial for stress reduction and weight management.

1. Somatic Breath Awareness

Somatic Breath Awareness is a practice that involves paying close attention to the breath and its effects on the body. It focuses on observing the breath without trying to change it, allowing individuals to become more aware of their breathing patterns and the sensations associated with breathing. This practice can help increase mindfulness, reduce stress, and promote relaxation

How To Do This: Sit or lie down in a comfortable position. Close your eyes and bring your attention to your breath pattern. Notice the natural rhythm of your breathing without trying to change it. Focus on the sensation of the breath entering and leaving your body.

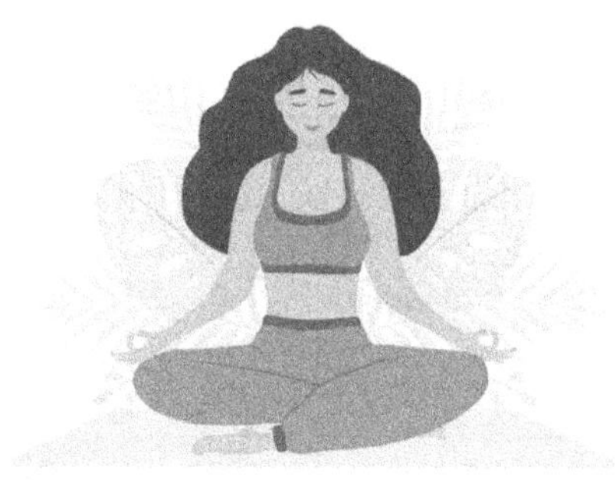

Duration: Practice for 5–10 minutes.

Repetition: there are no repetition, just concentrate on your breathing.

Benefits: Helps calm the mind, reduce stress, and improve focus and concentration.

2. Somatic Shoulder Stretch Release

Somatic Shoulder Stretch Release is a practice that involves gentle movements and techniques to release tension and pain in the shoulders. It aims to calm the body and mind by relieving excess tension. This practice can be beneficial for individuals experiencing shoulder stiffness, discomfort, or restricted range of motion

How To Do This: Sit or stand comfortably. Inhale, and as you exhale, gently roll your shoulders back and down, opening up the chest. Inhale and lift your shoulders towards your ears, then exhale and release them back down.

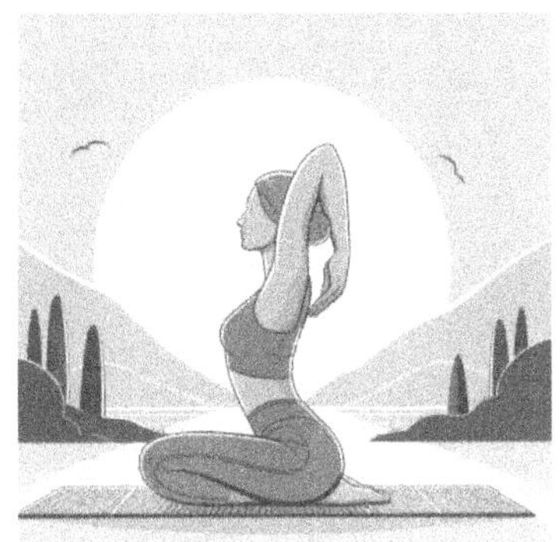 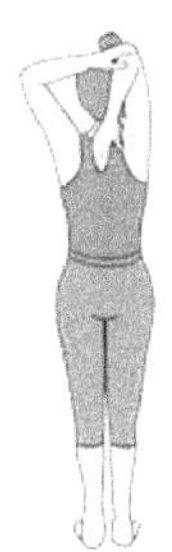

Repetitions: Repeat 5–8 times.

Duration: Practice for 1–3 minutes.

Benefits: Releases tension in the shoulders and upper back, and improves posture.

3. Somatic Forward Fold

A Somatic Forward Fold is a yoga pose that involves folding the upper body forward from the hips while standing, allowing the head to hang towards the ground. It's a gentle movement that aims to release tension in the back and hamstrings, improve flexibility, and promote relaxation. This pose can help calm the mind and reduce stress, making it a beneficial practice for overall well-being and body awareness.

How To Do This: Stand with your feet hip-width apart. Inhale and raise your arms overhead, then exhale and slowly fold forward from the hips, bending your knees slightly if needed. Let your head and arms hang towards the floor. Please refer to the diagram of Forward pose above to see illustration.

Repetitions: Repeat 2–3 times.

Duration: Hold a position for 30–60 seconds.

Benefits: Stretches the hamstrings and lower back, and calms the mind.

4. Somatic Seated Twist

Somatic Seated Twist is a yoga pose that involves sitting on the floor with legs extended and then twisting the upper body to one side, using the arms for support. This pose helps improve posture, flexibility, and digestion. It can also help release tension in the spine, shoulders, and neck, promoting relaxation and a sense of well-being

How To Do This: Sit on the floor with your legs extended in front of you. Bend your right knee and place your right foot on the outside of your left knee. Inhale and lengthen your spine, then exhale and twist to the right, placing your left elbow on the outside of your right knee. Hold for a few breaths, then repeat on the other side. Please refer to the Somatic Seated Twist diagram for illustration.

Repetitions: Repeat 3–5 times on each side.

Duration: Hold a position for 20–40 seconds.

Benefits: Improves digestion, massages the internal organs, reduces tension in the spine.

5. Somatic Legs-Up-The-Wall Pose

This is also known as Viparita Karani. It is a yoga pose where you lie on your back with your legs extended upward against a wall. This pose is believed to help improve circulation, reduce swelling in the legs, and promote relaxation by reversing the effects of gravity on the body. It is often used as a restorative pose to relieve stress and fatigue, and it can also help calm the mind and improve sleep quality. The pose is typically held for several minutes, allowing the body to fully relax and reap the benefits of the gentle inversion

How To Do This: Lie on your back with your legs extended up against a wall, forming a 90-degree angle with your body. Rest your arms by your sides with your palms facing up. Close your eyes and relax into the pose.

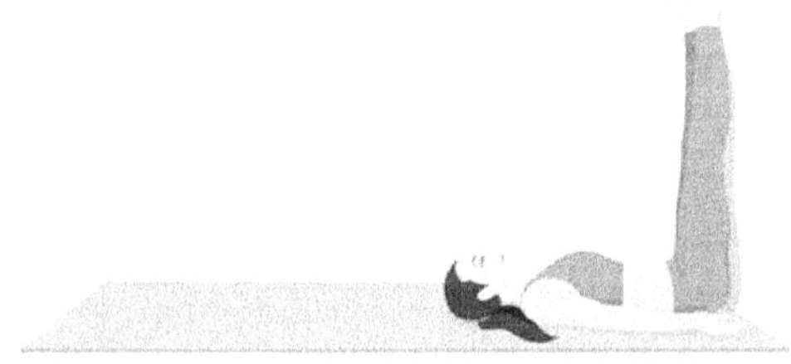

Duration: Hold for 10–20 minutes.

Benefits: Promotes relaxation, reduces stress and anxiety, and improves circulation.

6. Somatic Savasana (Corpse Pose)

This is a yoga pose that involves lying flat on the back with the arms and legs spread comfortably apart. It is typically practiced at the end of a yoga session to promote relaxation and rejuvenation. Somatic Savasana focuses on releasing tension from the body and calming the mind through deep breathing and mindfulness. This pose allows the body to integrate the benefits of the yoga practice, promoting a sense of peace and well-being

How To Do This: Lie on your back with your legs extended and your arms by your sides, palms facing up. Close your eyes and relax your entire body, letting go of any tension or stress.

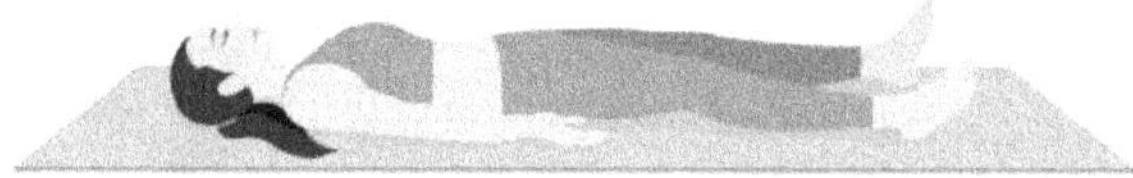

Duration: 10–20 minutes.

Benefits: Deeply relaxes the body and mind, and reduces stress and fatigue.

7. Somatic Full Body Relaxation

This involves a process of releasing tension and stress from the entire body using somatic therapy techniques. This approach focuses on increasing body awareness and promoting relaxation through mindful attention to physical sensations. It often includes practices such as progressive muscle relaxation, breathing exercises, and guided meditation to help individuals achieve a state of deep relaxation.

How To Do This: Lie on your back with your arms by your sides, palms facing up. Close your eyes and take deep, slow breaths. Starting from your toes, tense and then release each muscle group, working your way up to your head. Focus on relaxing each part of your body completely.

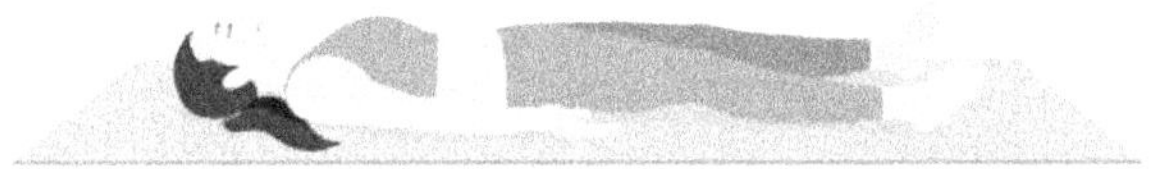

Repetitions: 1–2 times.

Duration: 5–15 minutes.

Benefits: Promotes deep relaxation, reduces muscle tension, reduces anxiety, improves sleep quality, enhances overall well-being, and calms the mind.

8. Somatic Child's Pose (Balasana)

The child pose also known as Balasana, is a yoga pose that helps to release tension and promote relaxation by gently stretching the hips, thighs, and ankles. It is a resting pose that is often used in yoga practice to calm the mind, relieve stress, and fatigue. Child's Pose can also help to alleviate back and neck pain by gently stretching the spine and relieving pressure on the lower back.

How To Do This: Kneel on the floor, sitting back on your heels. Slowly lower your torso forward, bringing your forehead to rest on the floor and extending your arms forward. Relax your entire body, focusing on deep breathing.

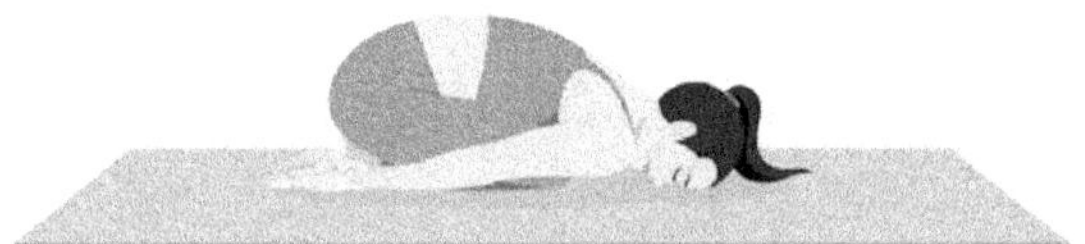 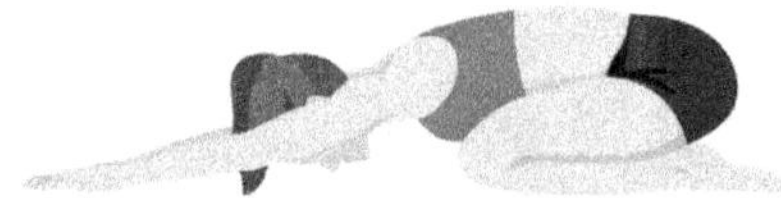

Repetitions: 1–3 times.

Duration: 2–5 minutes

Benefits: Stretches the spine, hips, and thighs, calms the mind, and relieves stress and fatigue. Also, great for increasing body awareness and promoting a sense of inner calm and relaxation

Practical Demonstration

To practice these poses, find a quiet space where you can relax without distractions.

Focus on your breath and move slowly and mindfully through each pose, paying attention to how your body feels.

Practice regularly to experience the full benefits of Somatic Yoga for stress reduction and weight management.

Somatic Yoga Sequences for Weight Loss

Somatic yoga sequences for weight loss refer to a combination of poses that work together to promote relaxation, improve flexibility, and reduce body fat. These are yoga poses that are based on the concept of somatic movement, which involves connecting the mind, body, and spirit through movement.

Although Somatic Yoga Exercises alone likely won't lead to significant weight loss, they can be an effective tool for your weight loss journey, because they help to reduce stress hormones that contribute to weight gain, improve sleep, and increase focus. Somatic yoga can also help to reduce inflammation, improve digestion, and reduce the risk of chronic diseases such as diabetes and heart disease.

Some examples of somatic yoga poses for weight loss include the downward dog, mountain pose, tree pose, warrior II, and cat-cow pose. These poses help to strengthen the core, stretch the joints and muscles, and improve balance and coordination.

1. Somatic Downward Dog (Adho Mukha Svanasana)

Somatic Downward Dog, or Adho Mukha Svanasana, is a yoga pose that combines stretching and strength-building. It is a foundational yoga pose that can be modified to suit different levels of flexibility and strength. It's a great pose for building overall body awareness and improving circulation.

How To Do This: Place your hands flat on the floor and your feet firm on the floor, lift your hips up and back, forming an inverted V shape. Press your hands and feet into the ground.

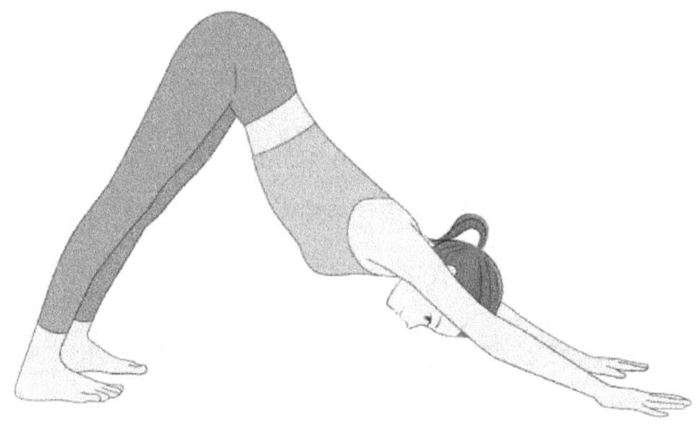

Duration: Hold for 30–60 seconds.

Repetitions: 3–5 times, with a few breaths of rest in between.

Benefits: Somatic Downward Dog stretches the hamstrings, calves, and shoulders, while also strengthening the arms and legs. It helps improve posture, relieve back pain, and calm the mind.

2. Somatic Mountain Pose (Tadasana)

Somatic Mountain Pose, also known as Tadasana, is a foundational yoga pose that focuses on alignment and grounding. It is a simple yet powerful pose that can help you connect with your body and find stability and strength both physically and mentally.

How To Do This: Stand tall with feet hip-width apart, arms relaxed by your sides. Engage your leg muscles and lengthen through your spine.

For Seated Pose: Sit comfortably with feet flat, spine aligned, sit bones grounded, and legs at a 90-degree angle. Relax shoulders, engage core, breathe deeply, lengthen neck, and focus on your breath to promote relaxation.

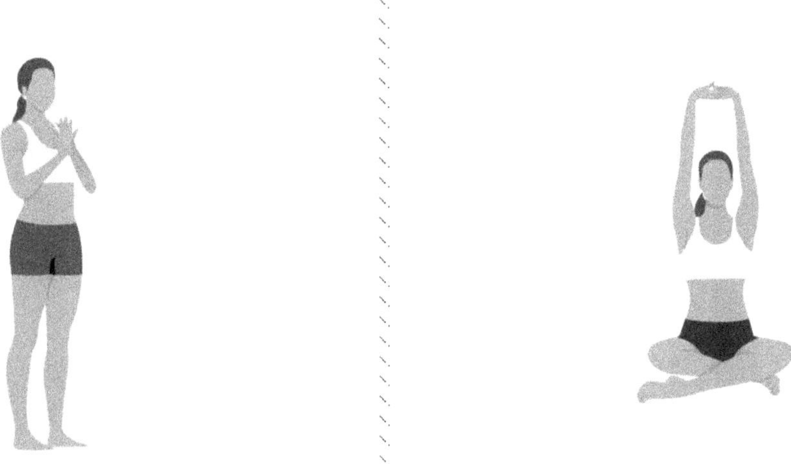

Duration: Hold for 30–60 seconds.

Repetitions: Repeat 5–10 times, focusing on alignment and breathing.

Benefits: Mountain Pose improves posture, strengthens thighs, knees, and ankles, and firms abdomen and buttocks. It also helps to reduce flat feet and can relieve sciatica.

3. Somatic Tree Pose (Vrksasana)

Somatic Tree Pose, is a grounding yoga pose that enhances concentration, stability, and body alignment. It cultivates a sense of calmness and empowerment, aiding in finding balance both physically and mentally. By practicing Somatic Tree Pose regularly, you can improve your posture, strengthen your legs and core muscles, and develop a greater sense of self-awareness. This pose is not only beneficial for the body but also for the mind, as it encourages focus and inner strength.

How to do This: Start in Mountain Pose (Tadasana), shift your weight onto one foot, and lift the other foot to place it on the inner thigh, calf, or ankle of the standing leg. Avoid placing the foot on the knee. Press the foot and thigh together while lengthening the spine and reaching the arms overhead, palms together.

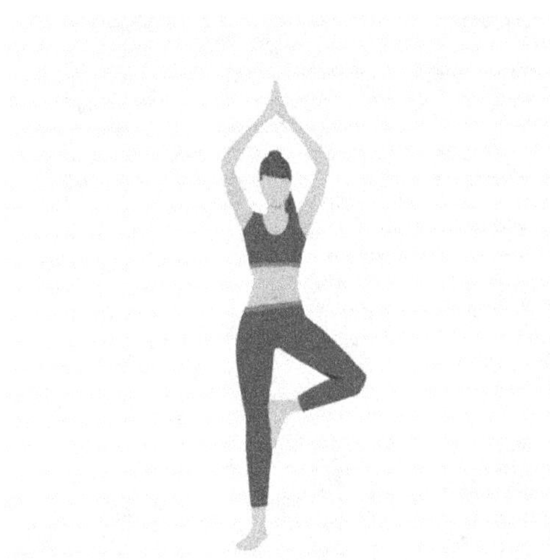

Duration: Hold for 20–40 seconds.

Repetitions: 3–5 times on each side, focusing on balance and stability.

Benefits: Tree Pose strengthens the legs, ankles, and core muscles. It improves balance, concentration, and body awareness.

4. Somatic Warrior II (Virabhadrasana II)

Somatic Warrior II, is a dynamic yoga pose that strengthens the legs, opens the hips, and improves focus. Warrior II helps cultivate stability, endurance, and mental resilience, making it a valuable posture for building strength and concentration in yoga practice.

How To Do This: From a standing position, step one foot back, rotate it 90 degrees, bend the front knee, and extend arms parallel to the floor.

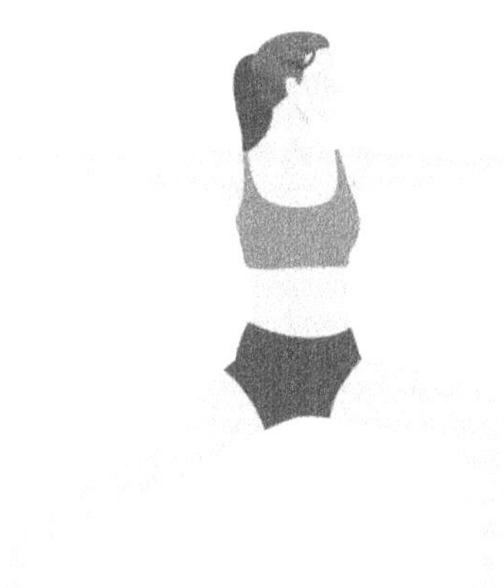

Duration: 20–40 seconds on each side.

Repetitions: Repeat 3–5 times on each side.

Benefits: Somatic Warrior II, or Virabhadrasana II, enhances balance, strength, and flexibility by targeting the legs, hips, core, and arms, while also improving stability and posture. Practicing this pose can cultivate concentration and focus, benefiting both physical and mental well-being.

5. The Somatic Bow Pose

Somatic Bow Pose, also known as Dhanurasana in traditional yoga, is a backbend posture that offers a deep stretch to the back and opens up the chest and shoulders. This pose helps improve flexibility, opens the heart center, and stimulates the digestive organs. It's a wonderful way to connect with your body and enhance your mind-body awareness1

How to Do This: Lie face down on your mat with your legs extended and arms resting by your sides.Bend your knees and bring your heels towards your buttocks. Reach back with your hands to grasp your ankles. Inhale deeply and lift your chest and thighs off the ground simultaneously. Use your hands to gently pull your ankles, deepening the stretch in your back.

Hold: Maintain this pose while breathing deeply, focusing on keeping your body relaxed and engaged. Exhale and slowly lower your chest and thighs back to the ground. Release your ankles and return to the starting position.

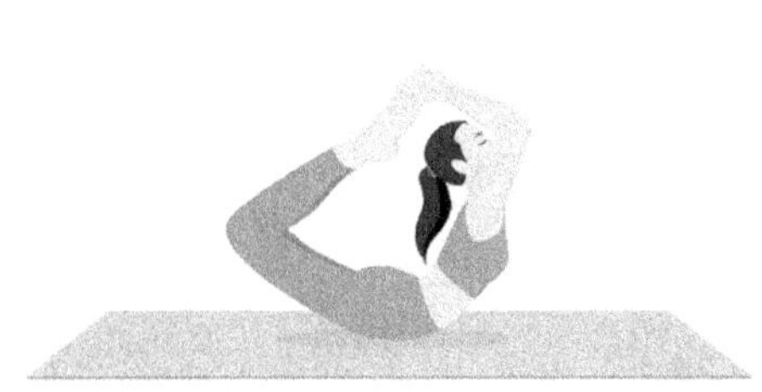
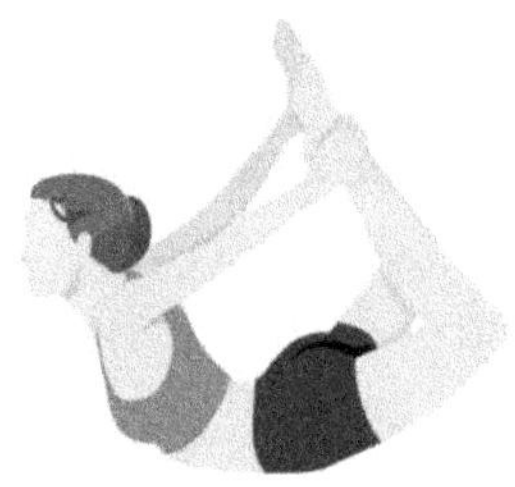

Duration: Hold each pose for 15-30 seconds.

Repetition: 2-3 times, with a short rest between.

Benefits:

- Strengthens the muscles in the back, helping to improve posture.
- Stretches the entire front body, including the chest, abdomen, and thighs, increasing overall flexibility.
- Releases tension in the shoulders and spine, promoting relaxation and stress relief.
- Stimulates blood flow throughout the body, contributing to overall vitality and well-being.

6. Somatic Bridge Pose

The Somatic Bridge Pose is a gentle backbend that releases tension in the lower back and abdominals, strengthens the core and glutes, and improves flexibility in the spine and hips. This pose also promotes better circulation and overall relaxation.

How To Do This: Lie on your back with your knees bent and feet flat on the floor, hip-width apart. Place your arms by your sides, palms facing down. Press your feet and arms into the ground. Inhale deeply. As you exhale, slowly lift your hips towards the ceiling, creating a straight line from your shoulders to your knees. Keep your thighs and feet parallel. Maintain this position for 15-30 seconds, breathing deeply. Exhale and gently lower your hips back to the floor. You can refer to the diagram in Somatic Bridge Pose above for illustration

Repetition: 3-5 times with a short rest in between.

Duration: Hold each pose for 15 - 30 seconds

Benefits:

- Engages the core and gluteal muscles, enhancing strength and stability.
- Stretches the chest, neck, spine, and hips.
- Alleviates tension in the lower back and promotes spinal health.
- Encourages blood flow and energizes the body.

7. Somatic Chair Pose

The Somatic Chair Pose is a gentle yoga posture that can be performed while sitting in a chair. It involves raising your arms overhead and gently bending forward, which helps release tension in the shoulders and back, strengthens the core and improves flexibility. This pose is especially beneficial for those who spend long hours sitting, promoting better posture and relaxation.

How to Do This: Stand with your feet hip-width apart and arms by your sides. Inhale and raise your arms overhead, keeping them parallel with palms facing inward. As you exhale, bend your knees and lower your hips as if sitting back into a chair. Keep your back straight and knees behind your toes. Inhale to straighten your legs and return to the starting position.

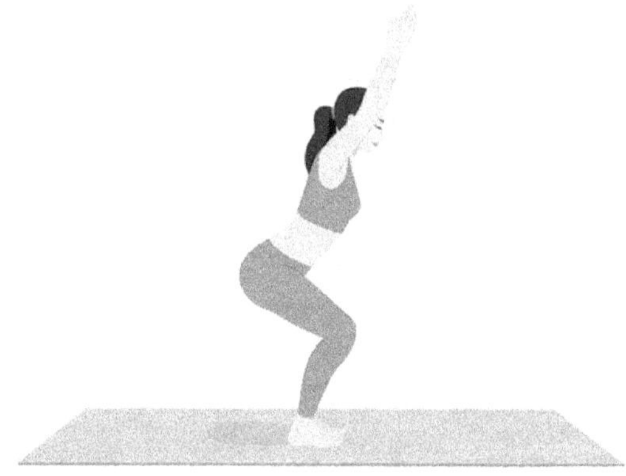

Duration: Hold position for 15-30 seconds, breathing deeply.

Repetition: 2-3 times with short rests in between.

Benefits:

- Engages the thighs, glutes, and core muscles, enhancing strength and endurance.
- Develops better balance and stability.

- Stretches the shoulders and chest.

- Enhances concentration and body awareness.

8. Somatic Revolved Triangle Pose (Trikonasana)

Somatic Trikonasana, also known as Revolved Triangle Pose, is a twisting yoga posture that provides a deep stretch to the spine and hamstrings. This pose enhances flexibility, improves balance, and strengthens the core, legs, and arms. Additionally, it promotes better circulation and helps relieve tension in the back and shoulders, making it an excellent choice for overall physical and mental well-being.

How to Do This: Stand with your feet about three to four feet apart. Turn your right foot out 90 degrees and your left foot slightly inwards. Raise your arms parallel to the floor, palms facing down. Inhale and extend your torso to the right, reaching your right hand down towards your shin or the floor, while your left arm extends upwards.

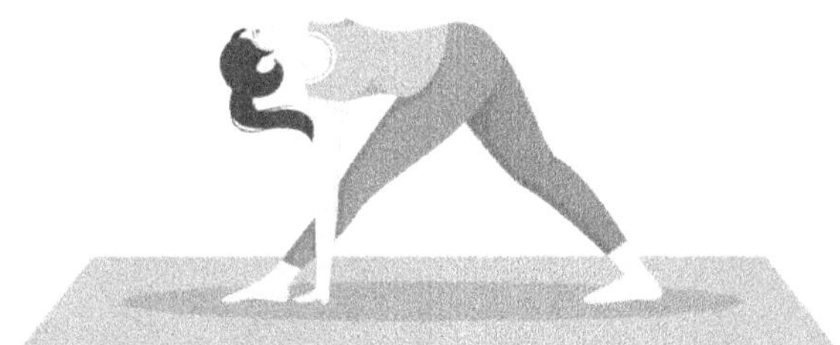

Duration: 15-30 seconds, breathing deeply.

Repetition: 2-3 times on each side.

Benefits:

- Enhances flexibility, stretches the legs, hips, and spine.

- Promotes better balance and stability.

- Strengthens muscles, engages the core, legs, and arms, building strength.

- Increases Circulation: Stimulates blood flow and revitalizes the body.

Practical Demonstration

To practice these yoga sequences, you should find a quiet space where you can move freely.

Focus on your breath and move slowly and mindfully through each pose, paying attention to how your body feels. Practice each sequence at least 3 times per week to see results.

Somatic Yoga Exercises for Emotion Balancing

Somatic Yoga can be a powerful tool for balancing emotions and promoting mental well-being. Emotional balance is essential for overall well-being and can greatly impact our physical health. Somatic Yoga offers gentle yet effective exercises to help balance emotions by releasing tension, calming the mind, and promoting relaxation.

In this section, we will focus on Somatic Yoga Exercises that are meant for releasing tension and stress held in the body, which can help to improve emotional stability and resilience. Practicing these exercises regularly can help you to feel more grounded, calm, and promote a sense of inner peace.

Some of these Somatic Yoga Poses like **Somatic Spinal Twist, Somatic Child's Pose, Somatic Butterfly Stretch, Somatic Breath Awareness, Somatic Shoulder Release** have already been covered in our previous sections. Kindly refer to them if you want to perform any of the pose.

Now, let's look at others that make up the list of Somatic Yoga Poses for emotional balancing

1. Somatic Body Scan

A Somatic Body Scan is a type of meditation practice where you focus your attention on different parts of your body, one by one, noticing physical sensations without judgment. It's a way to increase body awareness and relaxation, and can be used to manage stress, anxiety, and chronic pain

How To Do This: Lie down on your back with your arms by your sides, palms facing up. Close your eyes and bring your awareness to your body. Starting from your toes, bring your attention to each body part, noticing any tension or discomfort. Take a deep breath in, and as you exhale, release any tension you are holding in that body part. Continue scanning your body, releasing tension with each exhale.

Duration: Practice for 10–30 minutes.

Benefits: Promotes relaxation, releases physical and emotional tension, improves body awareness.

2. Somatic Twist

Somatic Twist is a movement that involves rotating the body to gently stretch and release tension in the muscles, particularly in the spine, neck, and shoulders. This practice aims to increase flexibility, improve posture, and promote relaxation by engaging in slow, deliberate movements and conscious breathing. You can use this move to reset muscle length and tension levels, improving your physical and mental well-being.

How To Do This: Sit on the floor with your legs extended in front of you. Bend one knee and cross it over the opposite leg, placing the foot flat on the floor. Place the opposite elbow on the outside of the bent knee and gently twist your torso towards the bent knee. Hold for a few breaths, then switch sides.

Other Twists: You can also include other somatic twisted pose in this session. Such as the Spinal Twist.

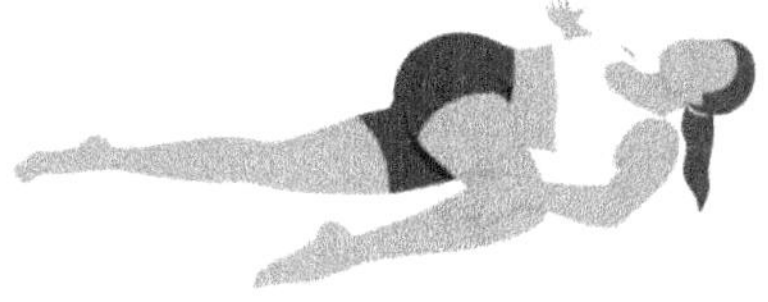

The Spinal Twist

Duration: 15–30 seconds

Repetitions: 3–5 on each side.

Benefits: Stretches the spine and muscles along the torso, improves digestion, releases tension in the back.

5. Somatic Heart Opener

This particular Somatic Exercise focuses on releasing tension and opening up the chest area to promote emotional well-being and a sense of openness. It often involves gentle movements and breathing exercises to help you connect with your emotions and cultivate a sense of compassion and self-awareness. There are various types of somatic heart opener poses and they include: **Half Camel Pose, Bridge Pose, Camel Pose, Cobra Pose, Fish Pose**

How To Do This: See the illustration of the different poses below to learn how to perform each of the somatic heart opener pose

Fish Pose

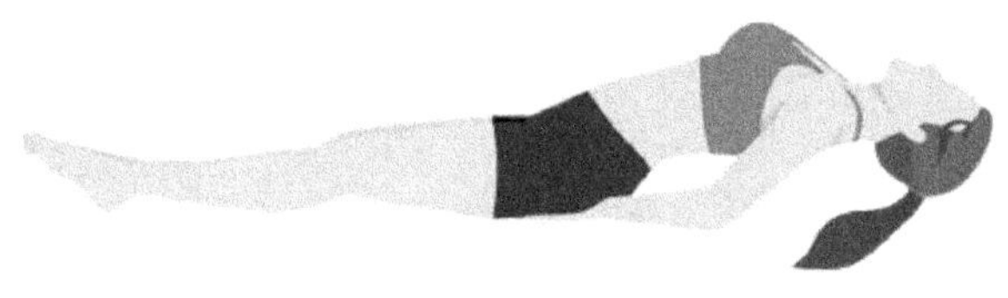

Half Camel Pose

Bridge Pose

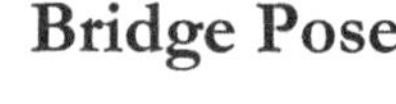

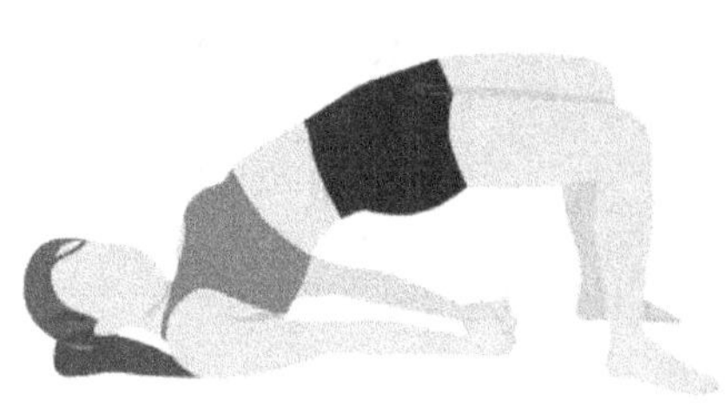

Camel Pose

Cobra Pose

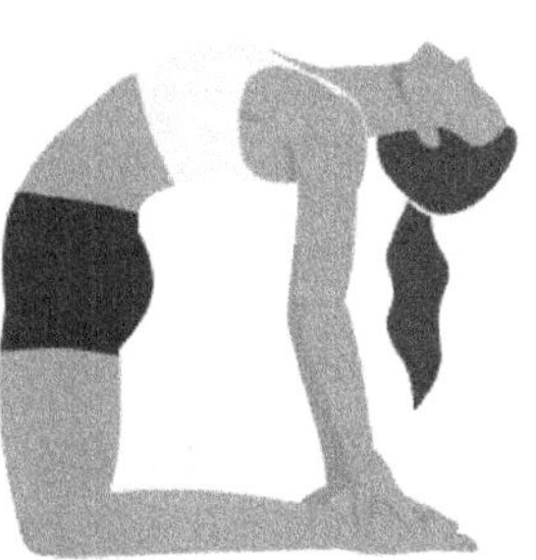

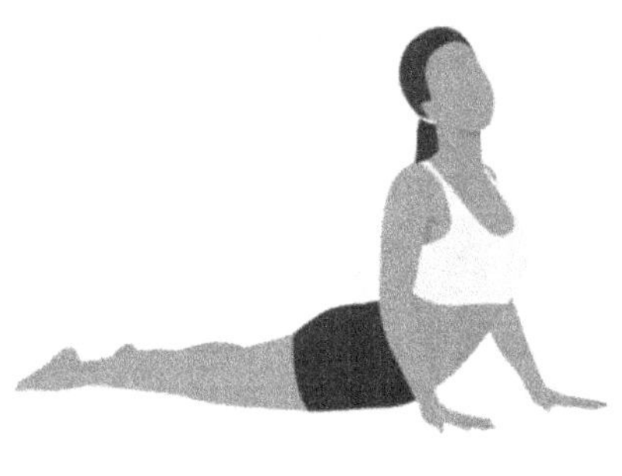

Duration: Hold for 15–30 seconds.

Repetition: 3–5 times

Benefits: Improves posture, opens the chest and shoulders, promotes emotional release.

Practical Demonstration

To practice these poses, you need to find a quiet space where you can relax without distractions.

Focus on your breath and move slowly and mindfully through each exercise, paying attention to how your body and emotions respond.

Practice regularly to maintain emotional balance and promote overall well-being.

Note: It's important to listen to your body and practice these exercises mindfully. If you have any medical conditions or injuries, kindly consult with your doctor or a healthcare professional before starting any new exercise program.

Somatic Yoga Restorative Poses

Somatic Yoga Restorative Poses focus on deep relaxation and rejuvenation. These poses are designed to release tension, calm the mind, and promote overall well-being. They are often held for longer periods, allowing the body to fully relax and release stress. Practicing these poses regularly can help reduce anxiety, improve sleep quality, and enhance overall health.

1. Supported Child's Pose

The Supported Child's Pose, also known as Salamba Balasana, is a restorative yoga posture that provides a gentle stretch to the back and hips while promoting relaxation and stress relief. Here's how you can perform it:

How To Do This: Begin by kneeling on your yoga mat with your knees hip-width apart and your big toes touching. Gently fold forward from your hips, extending your torso over your thighs. Allow your forehead to come to rest on the mat.

Adding Support: To make this a supported pose, place a bolster or a folded blanket between your thighs and your torso. This provides a cushion for your body to relax into, making the pose more comfortable and restorative.

Arm Placement: Your arms can be extended in front of you with palms facing down, or they can be relaxed alongside your body with palms facing up.

Breathing: Once in position, close your eyes and focus on taking deep, slow breaths. Inhale and exhale through your nose, allowing each breath to deepen your relaxation.

Duration: 5–10 minutes.

Repetitions: Hold the pose without repetitions.

Benefits:

- Relieves tension in the back, shoulders, and neck.

- Calms the mind and helps reduce stress and anxiety.

- Gently stretches the hips, thighs, and ankles.

- Encourages a sense of safety and comfort, as the pose is grounding and nurturing.

2. Grounding Spinal Twist

The Somatic Grounding Spinal Twist is a gentle, restorative yoga pose that involves a twisting motion of the spine to release tension and promote relaxation. It's part of the somatic movement practices, which focus on the internal experience of movement to enhance the mind-body connection.

How To Do This: Lie flat on your back on a comfortable surface, with your arms extended to the sides in a 'T' shape for stability. Bring your knees toward your chest, then gently lower them to one side, keeping your shoulders flat on the ground.

Deepening the Twist: Turn your head to look in the opposite direction of your knees to deepen the twist along the spine.

Breathing: Take deep, slow breaths, allowing each exhale to help you relax deeper into the twist.

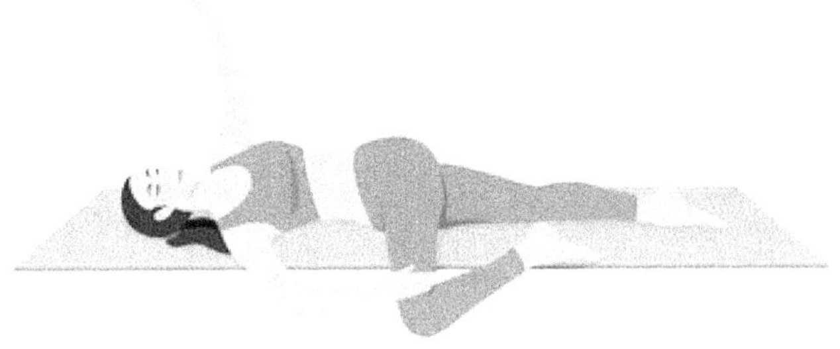

Duration: Hold the twist for 3–5 minutes on each side to allow your body to fully relax and release.

Repetitions: There are no repetitions needed; the focus is on holding the pose and experiencing the gentle release.

Benefits:

- Releases tension along the spine, which can help alleviate back pain.
- Promotes relaxation of the nervous system, which can reduce stress and anxiety.
- Stimulates digestion by massaging the abdominal organs.
- Improves flexibility and mobility in the spine and back muscles.

3. Head to Bolster Pose/ Supported Child Pose

The Somatic Head to Bolster Pose is a restorative yoga position that involves resting the head on a bolster or cushion to promote relaxation and improve breathing. This pose is suitable for anyone looking to unwind and connect with their body, especially after a long day or a strenuous activity. It's a simple yet effective way to introduce restorative practices into your yoga routine. Remember to adjust the position to ensure maximum comfort and to avoid any strain on your body.

How To Do This: Sit comfortably on your yoga mat with your legs crossed or in a position that feels natural for you. Place a yoga bolster or a folded blanket horizontally in front of you. Gently hinge forward from your hips and lay your forehead on the bolster, allowing your head to be fully supported.

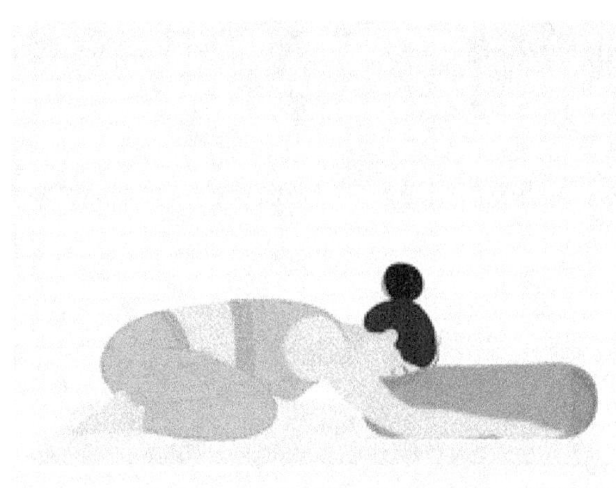

Arm Placement: Your arms can either rest by your sides or be stretched out in front of you, whichever feels more relaxing.

Breathing: Close your eyes and focus on taking deep, slow breaths. Feel the rise and fall of your chest and abdomen as you breathe.

Duration: 5–10 minutes,

Repetitions: No repetitions needed; the aim is to maintain the position and allow yourself to relax into the support of the bolster.

Benefits:

- Improves breathing rhythm by resting the head
- Activates the parasympathetic nervous system that helps to calm the mind and body, reducing stress and promoting a sense of well-being.
- Help relieve tension in the neck region.

4. Surfboard Pose

The Somatic Surfboard Pose is a restorative yoga pose designed to release tension in the lower back, sacrum, and shoulders while promoting relaxation and grounding. It's a variation of the traditional Surfboard Pose, also known as Salamba Salabhasana or Supported Locust Pose. This is a gentle way to soothe the body and mind, making it a valuable addition to your restorative yoga practice.

How To Do This: Lie face down on your mat with your arms extended alongside your body, palms facing down. Place a folded blanket or bolster under your hips and abdomen for support. Inhale and lift your chest, arms, and legs off the ground, keeping your neck in line with your spine. Maintain this position for 15-30 seconds, breathing deeply. Exhale and slowly lower your chest, arms, and legs back to the ground.

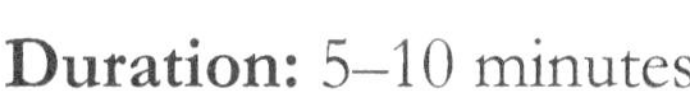

Duration: 5–10 minutes

Repetitions: No repetitions needed

Benefits:

- Releases tension in the sacrum and lower back.
- Relieves stiffness in the neck, upper back, and shoulders.
- Promotes relaxation and can be calming for those feeling anxious or overwhelmed.
- Stimulates the digestive system and kidneys due to the prone position.

Caution: If you have eye problems, lower back issues, or a pacemaker, you should modify the pose or consult with a healthcare professional before attempting it.

5. Supported Bridge Pose

The Somatic Supported Bridge Pose, also known as Salamba Setu Bandhasana, is a gentle variation of the traditional Bridge Pose. However, this uses props to provide support, allowing for a more restorative experience.

How To Do This: Lie on your back on a yoga mat with your knees bent and feet flat on the floor, hip-width apart. Press your feet into the floor to lift your hips up.

Adding Support: Slide a yoga block or bolster under your sacrum, which is the triangular bone at the base of your spine. Ensure the support is stable and comfortable.

Arm Position: Extend your arms along the floor, palms facing down, or you can place them on your belly to connect with your breath.

Allow your body to relax into the support, letting gravity gently open up the front of your hips and the spine.

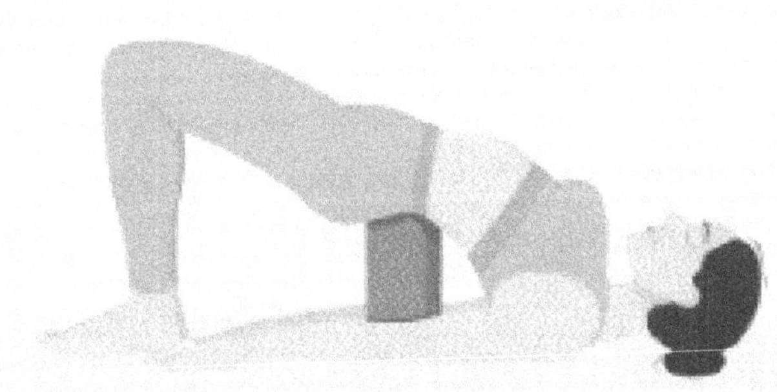

Duration: 5–10 minutes

Repetition: No repetitions needed

Benefits

- Extends the spine, which can alleviate back pain and improve posture.

- Promotes relaxation and activates the parasympathetic nervous system.

- Helps open the chest for better breathing and counteracts the hunch from poor posture.

- Tones the organs in the pelvis and abdomen, and puts gentle pressure on the lower back.

- Increases blood flow through the neck and throat, which can be rejuvenating.

6. Supported Fish Pose

Supported Fish Pose, known as Matsyasana in Sanskrit, is a restorative yoga pose and a gentle backbend pose type that opens up the chest and throat, promotes spinal flexibility, and can help alleviate respiratory ailments.

How To Do This: Sit on the floor with your legs extended in front of you.

Place a yoga block or bolster horizontally behind you where your shoulder blades will rest.

Slowly recline your torso back over the block or bolster, ensuring it supports your mid-back and shoulder blades. Allow your head to tilt backward and rest on the floor, if comfortable.

Extend your arms out to the sides at a 45-degree angle, palms facing up. Keep your legs relaxed and either extended or in a cross-legged position.

Duration: 1–5 minutes

Repetition: 1–3 times

Benefits:

- Increases spinal flexibility and improves posture.

- Opens the chest and helps to relieve the tightness, beneficial for respiratory issues.

- Stretches the neck and shoulders, which can be soothing if you spend a lot of time at a desk.

- Activates the Throat Chakra (Vishuddha), Heart Chakra (Anahata), and Solar Plexus Chakra (Manipura), which may help in improving communication, emotional balance, and personal power.

- Relieves stress and tension by promoting relaxation and deep breathing.

7. Heart Pose with Butterfly Legs

The Somatic Heart Pose with Butterfly Legs is a restorative yoga pose that combines the heart-opening aspect of a back bend with the hip-opening benefits of the butterfly legs position.

How To Do The: Begin by sitting on the floor with a bolster or a stack of folded blankets behind you. Bring the soles of your feet together, allowing your knees to fall out to the sides, forming the butterfly legs position.

Slowly lean back onto the bolster or blankets, ensuring that your spine is supported from the sacrum to the head. Let your arms rest by your sides or place them on your belly or heart, whichever feels more comfortable.

Close your eyes and focus on your breath, inhaling deeply through the nose and exhaling slowly through the mouth.

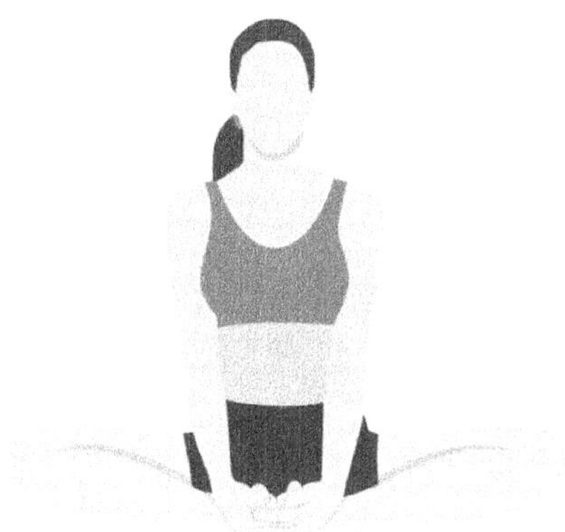

Duration: 5 to 20 minutes

Repetition: No repetitions, just hold the pose and allow your body to relax and settle into the position.

Benefits:

- Encourages emotional release and enhances feelings of compassion and love.
- Helps release tension in the hips, which can be beneficial for those who sit for long periods.
- Stimulates the parasympathetic nervous system*
- Improves circulation in the heart and lungs.
- Enhances breathing

8. Gentle Spinal Twist

The Somatic Gentle Spinal Twist is a calming yoga pose that focuses on releasing tension in the spine and promoting relaxation throughout the body. It involves slow, mindful twisting of the spine while focusing on the sensations within the body.

How To Do This: Sit on the floor with your legs extended in front of you.

Bend your right knee and place the sole of your right foot on the outside of your left knee.

Inhale to lengthen your spine upwards. As you exhale, gently twist your torso to the right, placing your left hand on your right knee and your right hand behind you for support.

Hold the twist for a few breaths, then release and repeat on the opposite side.

Remember to move into and out of the twist slowly and mindfully, paying attention to how your body feels and making any necessary adjustments to ensure comfort and safety.

Duration: 30 seconds to 1 minute on each side.

Repetition: 2–3 times on each side

Benefits:

- Helps to alleviate stiffness and discomfort in the back.
- Encourages the release of stress and can be soothing for the nervous system.
- The twisting motion can stimulate digestive organs and enhance digestion
- Increases flexibility and mobility in the spine and back muscles.
- Encourages mindfulness and body awareness.

9. Basic Relaxation Pose

The Somatic Basic Relaxation Pose is a foundational practice in somatic yoga, designed to foster deep relaxation and re-establish the mind-body connection. It is a form of somatic exercise that focuses on the awareness of bodily sensations and the use of slow, deliberate movements to bring about a state of relaxation. This practice can help reduce stress, improve flexibility, and enhance overall well-being

How To Do This: Find a quiet, comfortable space where you won't be disturbed. Lie down on your back on a yoga mat or a soft surface.

Allow your legs to extend naturally, with a slight distance apart, and let your feet fall to their sides.

Place your arms alongside your body, palms facing up, to open your chest and shoulders.

Close your eyes and take a few deep breaths, inhaling through the nose and exhaling through the mouth.

Scan your body from head to toe, consciously releasing tension from each part.

Duration: Stay in the pose for 10 to 20 minutes

Repetition: No repetitions, just practice at the end of a yoga session or before bedtime to promote better sleep.

Benefits:

- By focusing on the breath and body sensations, it helps calm the mind, reduces stress and anxiety.
- Promotes relaxation by encouraging the muscles to release tension and the nervous system to enter a state of rest.
- Helps you become more attuned to the subtle cues of your body.
- Enhances sleep quality
- Restorative poses like this allow the body to activate its natural healing processes.

10. Reclining Bound Angle Pose (Supta Baddha Konasana)

This Yoga Pose is a gentle and relaxing stretch that targets the hips, inner thighs, and lower back. The pose helps open the hips and groin, stretches the inner thighs and knees, and can help alleviate menstrual discomfort and sciatica. It is often used for relaxation and to release tension in the lower body.

How To Do This: Lie on your back and bring the soles of your feet together, allowing your knees to fall open to the sides. Support your knees with blocks or cushions if needed.

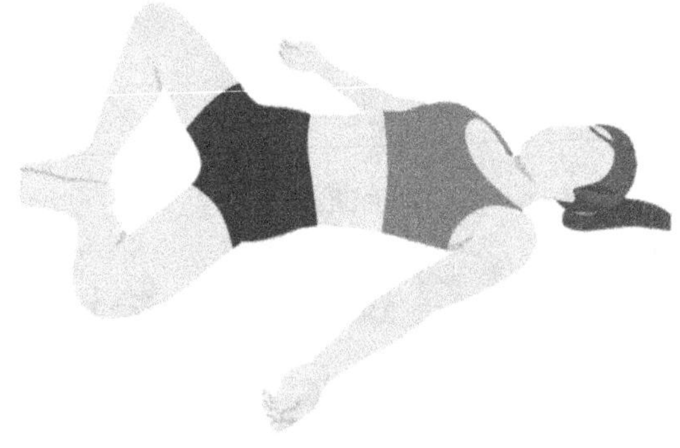

Duration: Hold for 3–5 minutes.

Repetition: 2–4 times

Benefits:

- Opens the hips and groin.

- Relieves menstrual discomfort and mild depression.

- Stretches the hips, inner thighs, and lower back.

- Calms the mind and body.

- Helps reduce lower back tension.

- Can improve digestion and relieve stress.

Practical Demonstration

To practice these poses, find a quiet space and gather any props you may need. Focus on your breath and allow yourself to relax deeply into each pose.

Hold each pose for the recommended duration, breathing deeply and evenly.

These poses can be practiced daily, especially if you're dealing with stress or seeking relaxation.

The best time for Somatic Yoga is when you can be undisturbed and relaxed, often before bed or upon waking.

Use props like bolsters, blankets, and blocks to support your body and encourage complete relaxation.

Note: *It's important to listen to your body and modify the poses as needed to suit your comfort level. If you have any medical conditions or injuries, consult with a healthcare professional before starting a new exercise program.*

Nutritional Tips to Complement Somatic Yoga Practice

Nutrition plays a crucial role in enhancing and complementing your somatic yoga practice. Somatic yoga focuses on internal experience and mindfulness, and integrating the right nutrition can significantly improve the benefits you receive from your practice. These nutritional practices plays a crucial role in complementing your somatic yoga practice by providing the body with the necessary nutrients for energy, flexibility, and overall health.

1. Hydration is Key: Staying well-hydrated is essential for any physical activity, including yoga. Water helps to keep the joints lubricated, aids in muscle recovery, and ensures that all bodily functions are running smoothly. Aim to drink plenty of water before and after your yoga sessions to maintain optimal hydration levels.

2. Mindful Eating: Somatic yoga encourages a deep connection with your body, and this can extend to how you eat. Practice mindful eating by paying attention to the flavors, textures, and sensations of your food. This can help you better understand your body's needs and responses to different foods.

3. Balanced Diet for Energy: A balanced diet that includes a mix of carbohydrates, proteins, and healthy fats will provide you with the sustained energy needed for your yoga practice. Carbohydrates are the body's primary energy source, while proteins support muscle repair and growth. Healthy fats are essential for hormone production and joint health.

4. Nutrient-Dense Foods for Recovery: After a somatic yoga session, it's important to replenish your body with nutrient-dense foods. These include fruits, vegetables, whole grains, nuts, seeds, and legumes. They provide the vitamins and minerals necessary for muscle recovery and overall well-being.

5. Anti-Inflammatory Foods: Incorporate anti-inflammatory foods into your diet to help reduce muscle soreness and support recovery. Foods rich in omega-3 fatty acids, like salmon, flaxseeds, and walnuts, can be particularly beneficial to your body.

6. Pre- and Post-Yoga Snacks: Consider having a small snack before your yoga practice to fuel your body. A combination of simple carbohydrates and protein, such as a banana with almond butter, can give you a quick energy boost. After yoga, a protein-rich snack can aid in muscle recovery.

7. Listen to Your Body: Each person's nutritional needs are unique, so it's important to listen to your body and adjust your diet accordingly. If you notice certain foods don't sit well with you before yoga, try to avoid them and see how you feel — this is a great way to keep your body healthy.

8. Timing of Meals: Be mindful of the timing of your meals in relation to your yoga practice. Eating a large meal right before yoga can be uncomfortable, so aim to have your main meal at least two hours before your session. A light snack 30 minutes before can be helpful if you need a little boost.

9. Supplements: If you're unable to get all the necessary nutrients from your diet alone, consider supplements. However, it's best to consult with a healthcare professional before adding any supplements to your routine.

10. Avoid Processed Foods: Minimize the intake of processed foods, which can be high in sugar and unhealthy fats. These can lead to energy crashes and are not conducive to the mindful, holistic approach of somatic yoga.

By following these nutritional tips, you can create a diet that will greatly fuel your somatic yoga practice and also contributes to your overall health and well-being.

Remember, the goal is to nourish your body in a way that supports the connection and awareness you cultivate through somatic yoga.

Building a Sustainable Somatic Yoga Practice

Embarking on a weight loss journey involves more than just shedding pounds—it's about fostering holistic well-being and creating sustainable habits. Integrating Somatic Yoga Exercises into your Weight Loss routine can be a powerful way to achieving long-lasting success.

Somatic yoga, with its focus on the internal experience of movement, can be a powerful tool for both shedding some pounds and improving overall well-being. Let's look at some of the benefits of Somatic Yoga Exercise for weight loss

Benefits of Somatic Yoga for Weight Loss

While somatic yoga is not a high-intensity workout, it contributes to weight loss by:

- **Enhancing body awareness:** Helps in recognizing hunger and fullness cues.

- **Reducing stress:** Helps in lowering stress levels which contributes to the decrease of cortisol. This has been linked to weight gain.

- **Improving mood:** A better mood can reduce emotional eating.

- **Increasing muscle tone:** Somatic Yoga involves gentle movements that can help in toning the body.

Building Your Practice

To build a sustainable somatic yoga practice for your weight loss journey, you should consider the following steps:

> ➢ **Start with Awareness**

Begin by becoming aware of your body and its sensations. Body scans and progressive muscle relaxation (PMR) are excellent starting points. These practices help you identify areas of tension and release them, which is crucial for a mindful practice.

> ➢ **Incorporate Gentle Movements**

Gentle somatic exercises, such as those found in the above, can release pent-up emotions and tension. These movements are typically slow and controlled, focusing on the quality of movement rather than the quantity.

> ➢ **Practice Regularly**

Consistency is key. Aim for a daily practice, even if it's just for a few minutes. Over time, this will help you develop a habit that supports weight loss and overall health.

> ➢ **Focus on Breathwork**

Breathwork is an integral part of somatic yoga. It helps to deepen the mind-body connection and supports relaxation and stress reduction.

➢ **Integrate Ideokinesis**

Ideokinesis is about visualizing and directing the flow of energy in the body. This can be particularly helpful in a weight loss journey as it encourages a positive and intentional approach to movement.

➢ **Focus on Core-Engaging Poses**

Engage in poses that target the core muscles: These poses have been mentioned above. Some of them includes

- **Plank:** Strengthens the abdominal muscles and improves digestion.
- **Boat Pose:** Further engages the core and promotes a healthy metabolism.
- **Twists:** Enhance digestion and aid in weight loss.

➢ **Embrace Mindful Eating Practices**

Yoga encourages mindfulness, which extends to your eating habits. You need to pay attention to taste and texture of what you eat, listen to your body and be able to recognize hunger and fullness cues. Avoid distractions during meals. — This mindful approach leads to healthier food choices.

➢ **Include Restorative Yoga for Stress Reduction**

Stress often contributes to weight gain. Incorporating restorative yoga sessions will help in your weight loss journey as well. We already covered the restorative yoga poses you can use earlier on this book. Go through them and incorporate them as you embark on your weight loss journey.

>Combine Yoga with Cardio and Strength Training

While Somatic Yoga offers numerous benefits, complementing it with other cardio exercises will greatly aid your weight loss journey.

Some cardiovascular activities you can incorporate includes: Walking, jogging, or cycling.

>Duration and Repetition

If you plan on incorporating Somatic Yoga poses into your weight loss journey, aim for practices that lasts at least 20-30 minutes. You can start with shorter sessions and gradually increase the duration as your body adapts.

>Set Intentional Goals

Align your weight loss goals with broader intentions such as:

- **Self-acceptance:** Embrace your journey.
- **Self-love:** Cultivate a positive mindset.
- **Gratitude:** Appreciate your body and progress.

>Seek Guidance

Consider seeking guidance from a qualified somatic yoga instructor who can tailor a practice to your needs and ensure that you're performing movements correctly.

Remember that sustainable weight loss involves patience, self-compassion, and a holistic approach.

Monitoring Progress: How to Track Weight Loss Journey with Somatic Yoga

Monitoring your progress during your weight loss journey is essential to stay motivated and make informed adjustments. When combining Somatic Yoga Exercise with weight loss goals, monitoring and tracking becomes even more valuable. In this session, let's explore how you can effectively monitor your progress:

- ➢ **Set Clear Goals:** Before you begin, define what success looks like for you. It could be a specific weight, how your clothes fit, or how you feel in your body.

- ➢ **Keep a Journal:** Document your Somatic Yoga practice and any changes you notice in your body or mood. Note the date, duration of practice, and any particular sensations or emotions that arise.

- ➢ **Take Measurements:** Use a tape measure to record the size of different body parts. Comparing measurements over time can show you where you're losing inches, even if the scale doesn't move.

- ➢ **Photographic Evidence:** Taking photos of yourself at regular intervals can be a powerful visual representation of your progress. Take photos of yourself at regular intervals (e.g., every month). Compare these photos to observe changes in body composition, posture, and muscle tone.

➢ **Mind-Body Connection:** Pay attention to how your body feels during and after Somatic Yoga sessions. Increased ease of movement, reduced pain, and a greater sense of relaxation can all be indicators of progress.

➢ **Consult with a Professional:** Work with a Somatic Yoga instructor or a healthcare provider to set realistic goals and ensure you're practicing safely.

➢ **Energy Levels and Sleep Quality:** Improved energy levels and better sleep quality are positive signs. Somatic exercises can indirectly support weight loss by reducing stress and promoting overall well-being.

➢ **Clothing Fit:** Notice how your clothes fit. Are they becoming looser? This is a tangible indicator of progress.

➢ **Be Patient and Consistent:** Weight loss is a gradual process, and Somatic Yoga is about tuning into your body's needs. Consistency in practice will yield the best results over time.

Weight loss is just one aspect of health. Somatic Yoga can also help improve flexibility, reduce stress, and enhance overall well-being. Celebrate all forms of progress and be kind to yourself on this journey.

Overcoming Plateaus in Weight Loss with Somatic Yoga

When practicing Somatic Yoga, you might encounter plateaus where progress seems to stall. Hitting a plateau in weight loss can be frustrating, but with Somatic Yoga practices, you are be equipped with tools that will help you overcome this challenge.

In this session, we will look at some of the best practices and strategies that can help you in breaking through weight loss plateaus and get even better results.

Understanding Plateaus: A weight loss plateau occurs when you no longer lose weight despite continuing with your exercise and diet regimen. It's a common part of the weight loss journey. Understanding weight loss plateaus will help you know when your progress is stalled and what to do to keep making progress.

Reevaluate Your Routine: Once you hit weight loss plateaus, you need to reevaluate your routine. To do this, check the for the following and apply to your routine…

- **Variety**: Our bodies adapt to repetitive movements. If you've been doing the same somatic yoga sequence for weeks, consider mixing it up. Try new poses, explore different flows, and challenge your muscles in fresh ways.
- **Intensity**: Gradually increase the intensity of your practice. Add more dynamic movements, hold poses longer, or incorporate faster transitions. This shocks your system and encourages progress.

Mindful Eating: This approach leads to healthier food choices. Pay attention to the kind of food you eat and how they affect your body.

- **Quality over Quantity**: Revisit your eating habits. Are you mindfully nourishing your body? Focus on nutrient-dense foods rather than empty calories.
- **Portion Control**: Even healthy foods can lead to weight loss plateaus if consumed excessively. Pay attention to portion sizes.

Hydration and Sleep: Hydration and quality sleep are other aspects you will need to check and ensure you are having enough of them.

- **Hydrate**: Dehydration can hinder weight loss. You should drink plenty of water throughout the day.
- **Prioritize Sleep**: Lack of sleep affects hormones related to hunger and metabolism. Aim for 7-9 hours of quality sleep each night.

Stress Management: Check your stress level and incorporate poses and routines that will help lower your stress level. Also, engage in restorative yoga.

- **Cortisol**: High stress levels elevate cortisol, which can lead to weight gain. Incorporate stress-reducing practices like meditation, deep breathing, or gentle somatic movements.
- **Restorative Yoga**: Engage in restorative poses to calm your nervous system and reduce stress.

Strength Training: You can engage in strength training exercises to support your weight lost journey.

- **Muscle Burns Calories**: Building lean muscle mass boosts your metabolism. Consider adding strength training sessions to your routine.

- **Body weight Exercises**: Combine somatic yoga with body weight exercises like squats, lunges, and push-ups.

Set New Goals: Sometimes, it is best to set new goals to support your weight loss journey.

- **Non-Scale Victories**: Shift your focus from the scale to other achievements. Celebrate improved flexibility, balance, or reduced stress.
- **Functional Goals**: Set goals related to daily life—like being able to carry groceries effortlessly or climb stairs without getting winded. Or performing things you weren't able to do before.

Mindset Shift: Your mindset plays a vital role in your weight loss journey and progress. You need to ensure that you have the right mindset as you continue on this journey.

- **Patience**: You need to be patient with yourself. Plateaus are temporary. Trust the process and stay positive and be patient.
- **Positive Affirmations**: Remind yourself of your progress and affirm your commitment to health.

Track Non-Scale Progress: If the scale is not making progress, track other aspect, such as energy level, and how your clothes fits

- **Energy Levels**: Notice if you feel more energetic or less fatigued.
- **Clothing Fit**: Pay attention to how your clothes fit, regardless of the number on the scale.
- **Body Awareness**: Continue body scans and mindfulness practices.

Consult a Professional: It may be time to sec a professional. If you apply everything and nothing is working, you should try to see a professional and see advice. You could See:

- **Yoga Instructor**: Seek guidance from a somatic yoga instructor. They can offer personalized modifications and insights to help you.
- **Nutritionist or Dietitian**: A professional dietitian can help fine-tune your diet and address any nutritional gaps.

Stay Consistent and Kind to Yourself: Most importantly, be kind to yourself and stay consistent.

- **Consistency**: Keep showing up on your mat. Consistent practice yields results.
- **Self-Compassion**: Weight loss isn't linear. Be kind to yourself during plateaus.

Weight loss is not linear, and plateaus are a natural part of the process. Embrace them as opportunities for growth and learning. Your body is adapting, and with persistence, you'll break through and continue toward your weight loss goals.

Incorporating Somatic Yoga into Your Daily Routine

Somatic yoga is a transformative practice that invites you into a deeper connection with your body, melding movement with mindfulness to unlock a profound sense of awareness and healing. In this part, we will explore how you can incorporate somatic yoga into your daily routine even if you work 9–5 and are too busy:

Understanding Somatic Yoga

By now, you understand that Somatic Yoga is about tuning into your body's innate wisdom. Prioritizing internal experience over external appearance, allowing you to release tension, restore balance, and move with greater ease and intention.

Unlike traditional yoga styles that focus on external alignment, somatic yoga encourages you to explore and transform your body from within.

This is not just about the physical poses; it's about deepening your relationship with your body and experiencing movement from the inside out.

Think of it as "embodied yoga," where the poses are not the ultimate goal but a starting point for your own exploration.

Mindful Movement Throughout the Day

Now that we know this, knowing how to apply this as a mindful movement throughout your day is the key to performing effective Somatic Yoga practice.

You can integrate somatic practices into your everyday life by taking short breaks throughout the day to practice mindful breathing and movement even if it is for 5 minutes.

Do some simple stretches, paying attention to the sensations in your body as you move, and even a few minutes of meditation can all be part of your somatic routine.

Somatic Movement for Posture and Pain Relief

Incorporate somatic movement to improve your posture and reduce chronic pain. By focusing on internal sensations, you'll develop greater body awareness and control.

Whether you're sitting at your desk, standing in line, or walking, pay attention to how your body moves. Adjust your posture and release tension as needed.

Embrace Intuitive Movement

Somatic techniques allow you to tap into intuitive movement impulses. Stay with these impulses until they naturally run their course.

The goal is to reach a state of release where you can tolerate feeling okay—sometimes harder than it sounds. Somatic yoga helps you reconnect with your body and soothe your nervous system.

Integration into Daily Life

The insights gained through a somatic approach to yoga can be applied beyond the mat. You can bring mindfulness practices and body awareness into your everyday activities.

Harnessing this mind-body connection enhances overall well-being and supports your somatic journey.

Maintaining Weight Loss Achieved through Somatic Yoga

Maintaining weight loss achieved through somatic yoga requires a balanced approach that includes continued practice, mindful eating, and lifestyle adjustments.

In this session, we will look at some key things you should do to maintain the result achieved:

- ➤ **Regular Practice:** Continue to incorporate somatic yoga into your routine to maintain muscle tone, flexibility, and overall well-being.

- ➤ **Mindful Eating:** Practice mindful eating by paying attention to your body's hunger and fullness cues. Choose whole, nutrient-dense foods and avoid processed foods and sugary drinks.

- ➤ **Physical Activity:** Combine somatic yoga with other forms of physical activity you enjoy, such as walking, swimming, or cycling, to maintain a healthy weight and improve fitness.

- ➤ **Stress Management**: Continue to manage stress through somatic exercises and relaxation techniques. Chronic stress can lead to weight gain, so it's important to find healthy ways to cope.

➢ **Support System:** Surround yourself with a supportive community that encourages healthy habits and provides motivation.

➢ **Self-Care:** Prioritize self-care activities that promote relaxation and reduce stress, such as meditation, massage, or spending time in nature.

➢ **Professional Guidance:** Consider working with a somatic yoga instructor or health coach to create a personalized maintenance plan and provide ongoing support.

By incorporating these strategies into your lifestyle, you can maintain the weight loss achieved through somatic yoga and live a healthy life.

Daily Mindful Meditations

Daily mindful meditations are a practice that involves setting aside time each day to focus on the present moment with openness, curiosity, and acceptance. They are a wonderful way to cultivate presence, reduce stress, and enhance overall well-being.

In this part, we will discuss some practices you can incorporate into your daily routine for your daily mindful meditation.

> **Schedule Regular Sessions:** Set aside a specific time each day for your meditation practice. Remember, consistency is key to establishing a habit. To do this effectively, you could set an alarm for a specific time to remind you of your mindful meditation.

> **Start with Short Sessions and Comfortable Posture:** If you are a beginner, starting with short sessions will ensure you stay true to the Somatic session and not give up. You could begin with 5–10 minutes and gradually increase the duration as you become more comfortable with the practice. You should also start with the more comfortable posts.

> **Find a Quiet Space:** Choose a peaceful environment where you can comfortably practice your Somatic Yoga routines without distractions.

> **Focus on Your Breath:** Pay attention to the sensation of breathing in and out. If your mind wanders, gently bring it back to your breath without judgment.

➢ **Body Scan Meditation:** Bring your attention to different parts of your body, starting from your toes and moving up to your head. Notice any sensations or areas of tension, and breathe into those areas to release tension.

➢ **Loving-Kindness Meditation:** Repeat phrases of loving-kindness for yourself and others. For example, "May I be happy, may I be healthy, may I be safe, may I live with ease."

➢ **Walking Meditation:** Take a mindful walk, focusing on each step and the sensations in your body as you move. Notice the sights, sounds, and smells around you without getting caught up in thoughts.

Setting An Achievable Goal

To set an achievable goal for your Somatic Yoga routine you need to create a clear, realistic, and motivating target that aligns with your personal aspirations and physical capabilities.

In this session, I have created a comprehensive guide to help you establish and reach your Somatic Yoga goals

Below are the steps you will need to take:

Step 1: Define Your Intentions: Start by asking yourself why you want to practice Somatic Yoga. Is it for stress relief, flexibility, muscle recovery, or weight loss? Your intention will guide your goal-setting process.

Step 2: Assess Your Current State: Evaluate your current physical condition, flexibility, strength, and any health concerns. This assessment will help you set goals that are challenging yet attainable.

Step 3: Set SMART Goals: Specific, **M**easurable, **A**chievable, **R**elevant, and **T**ime-bound goals are more likely to be successful. For example, "I will practice Somatic Yoga for 30 minutes every morning to improve my flexibility and reduce stress."

Step 4: Create a Structured Plan: Outline a routine that includes a variety of Somatic Yoga poses targeting different muscle groups. Incorporate nutrition tips, such as eating anti-inflammatory foods and staying hydrated, to complement your practice. Luckily for you, this have been covered in this book.

Step 5: Monitor Your Progress: Keep a yoga journal to track your practice, how you feel after each session, and any improvements in your flexibility, strength, or stress levels.

Step 6: Celebrate Milestones: Recognize and celebrate small achievements along the way. This will keep you motivated and committed to your Somatic Yoga journey.

Step 7: Reflect and Reassess: Regularly reflect on your practice and goals. As you grow in your Somatic Yoga journey, your goals may evolve. Reassess and set new targets as needed.

Step 8: Integrate Mindfulness: Incorporate mindfulness into your routine to enhance the somatic experience. This can help with emotional eating and cravings by creating a deeper connection with your body's needs.

Monitoring Your Progress — The Journal

Somatic Yoga Practice Journal

Name: _________________________________ / **Date:** _______________

Morning Reflection:

Mood upon waking: _______________________Physical sensations: _______________________

Intentions for today's practice: ____

Yoga Session

Time of Practice: _______________________

Poses Practiced:

1. Pose Name: _______________________ | Duration: _________ | Repetitions: _________

2. Pose Name: _______________________ | Duration: _________ | Repetitions: _________

3. Pose Name: _______________________ | Duration: _________ | Repetitions: _________

4. Pose Name: _______________________ | Duration: _________ | Repetitions: _________

5. Pose Name: _______________________ | Duration: _________ | Repetitions: _________

6. Pose Name: _______________________ | Duration: _________ | Repetitions: _________

Somatic Focus Areas:

☐ Neck and Shoulders | ☐ Spine and Back | ☐ Hips and Pelvis

☐ Legs and Feet | ☐ Arms and Hands | ☐ Full Body Integration

Breathing Techniques Used:

Technique: _______________________________________ | Duration: _____________

Post-Session Reflection

Physical Observations:

Flexibility improvements: ____

Strength improvements: ____

Stress level changes: ____

Emotional Observations:

Mood after practice: ____

Emotional shifts: ____

Nutrition:

Breakfast: ____________________________________/Calorie: _________

Snacks: ____________________________________/Calorie: _________

Lunch: ____________________________________/Calorie: _______

Dinner: ____________________________________/ Calorie: ______

Additional Notes:

____

____

____

____

____

Progress Tracking

Weight Tracking:

Weight today: _______________ | Goal weight: ____

Flexibility Tracking:

Forward bend reach: _________________________________ | Goal: ___________________________

Strength Tracking:

Hold time for core poses: _____________________________ | Goal: _________________________

Stress Management:

Stress level (1-10): _________________________________ | Goal: ___________________________

Overall Well-being (1-10): ____

Goals for Next Session

____

____

____

____

____

____

____

____

____

____

____

____

Somatic Yoga Practice Journal

Name: ____/ Date: ___________________

Morning Reflection:

Mood upon waking: ______________________________Physical sensations: ____________________________

Intentions for today's practice: ____

Yoga Session

Time of Practice: ______________________________

Poses Practiced:

1. Pose Name: ________________________________ | Duration: __________ | Repetitions: __________

2. Pose Name: ________________________________ | Duration: __________ | Repetitions: __________

3. Pose Name: ________________________________ | Duration: __________ | Repetitions: __________

4. Pose Name: ________________________________ | Duration: __________ | Repetitions: __________

5. Pose Name: ________________________________ | Duration: __________ | Repetitions: __________

6. Pose Name: ________________________________ | Duration: __________ | Repetitions: __________

Somatic Focus Areas:

☐ Neck and Shoulders | ☐ Spine and Back | ☐ Hips and Pelvis

☐ Legs and Feet | ☐ Arms and Hands | ☐ Full Body Integration

Breathing Techniques Used:

Technique: ____ | Duration: ____________

Post-Session Reflection

Physical Observations:

Flexibility improvements: ____

Strength improvements: ____

Stress level changes: ____

Emotional Observations:

Mood after practice: ____

Emotional shifts: ____

Nutrition:

Breakfast: ____/Calorie: _________

Snacks: ____/Calorie: _________

Lunch: ____/Calorie: ________

Dinner: ____/ Calorie: _______

Additional Notes:

____

____

____

____

____

Progress Tracking

Weight Tracking:

Weight today: _______________ | Goal weight: _______________________________________

Flexibility Tracking:

Forward bend reach: _________________________________ | Goal: _______________________

Strength Tracking:

Hold time for core poses: _______________________________ | Goal: ___________________

Stress Management:

Stress level (1-10): _________________________________ | Goal: _____________________

Overall Well-being (1-10): ____

Goals for Next Session

____

____

____

____

____

____

____

____

____

____

____

____

Somatic Yoga Practice Journal

Name: ____/ **Date:** __________________

Morning Reflection:

Mood upon waking: ________________________Physical sensations: ________________________

Intentions for today's practice: ____

Yoga Session

Time of Practice: ______________________

Poses Practiced:

1. Pose Name: ______________________ | Duration: _________ | Repetitions: _________

2. Pose Name: ______________________ | Duration: _________ | Repetitions: _________

3. Pose Name: ______________________ | Duration: _________ | Repetitions: _________

4. Pose Name: ______________________ | Duration: _________ | Repetitions: _________

5. Pose Name: ______________________ | Duration: _________ | Repetitions: _________

6. Pose Name: ______________________ | Duration: _________ | Repetitions: _________

Somatic Focus Areas:

☐ Neck and Shoulders | ☐ Spine and Back | ☐ Hips and Pelvis

☐ Legs and Feet | ☐ Arms and Hands | ☐ Full Body Integration

Breathing Techniques Used:

Technique: ______________________________________ | Duration: ____________

Post-Session Reflection

Physical Observations:

Flexibility improvements: ____

Strength improvements: ____

Stress level changes: ____

Emotional Observations:

Mood after practice: ____

Emotional shifts: ____

Nutrition:

Breakfast: _____________________________________/Calorie: _________

Snacks: _______________________________________/Calorie: _________

Lunch: ____/Calorie: _______

Dinner: _______________________________________/ Calorie: ______

Additional Notes:

____

____

____

____

____

Progress Tracking

Weight Tracking:

Weight today: _______________ | Goal weight: ____

Flexibility Tracking:

Forward bend reach: ________________________________ | Goal: ____________________________

Strength Tracking:

Hold time for core poses: ____________________________ | Goal: ____________________________

Stress Management:

Stress level (1-10): ________________________________ | Goal: ____________________________

Overall Well-being (1-10): ____

Goals for Next Session

____
____
____
____
____
____
____
____
____
____
____

Somatic Yoga Practice Journal

Name: _______________________________________/ Date: ___________________

Morning Reflection:

Mood upon waking: _______________________Physical sensations: ___________________________

Intentions for today's practice: ____

Yoga Session

Time of Practice: _______________________________

Poses Practiced:

1. Pose Name: _________________________________ | Duration: ___________ | Repetitions: ___________

2. Pose Name: _________________________________ | Duration: ___________ | Repetitions: ___________

3. Pose Name: _________________________________ | Duration: ___________ | Repetitions: ___________

4. Pose Name: _________________________________ | Duration: ___________ | Repetitions: ___________

5. Pose Name: _________________________________ | Duration: ___________ | Repetitions: ___________

6. Pose Name: _________________________________ | Duration: ___________ | Repetitions: ___________

Somatic Focus Areas:

☐ Neck and Shoulders | ☐ Spine and Back | ☐ Hips and Pelvis

☐ Legs and Feet | ☐ Arms and Hands | ☐ Full Body Integration

Breathing Techniques Used:

Technique: ____ | Duration: ___________

Post-Session Reflection

Physical Observations:

Flexibility improvements: ____

Strength improvements: ____

Stress level changes: ____

Emotional Observations:

Mood after practice: ____

Emotional shifts: ____

Nutrition:

Breakfast: _______________________________________/Calorie: ________

Snacks: _______________________________________/Calorie: ________

Lunch: _______________________________________/Calorie: ________

Dinner: _______________________________________/ Calorie: ______

Additional Notes:

____

____

____

____

____

Progress Tracking

Weight Tracking:

Weight today: _______________ | Goal weight: ____

Flexibility Tracking:

Forward bend reach: ________________________________ | Goal: _______________________________

Strength Tracking:

Hold time for core poses: _______________________ | Goal: _______________________________

Stress Management:

Stress level (1-10): _______________________________ | Goal: _______________________________

Overall Well-being (1-10): ____

Goals for Next Session

____
____
____
____
____
____
____
____
____
____
____

Somatic Yoga Practice Journal

Name: ______________________________________/ **Date:** _________________________

Morning Reflection:

Mood upon waking: ________________________________Physical sensations: _______________________

Intentions for today's practice: ____

Yoga Session

Time of Practice: _______________________________

Poses Practiced:

1. Pose Name: _________________________________ | Duration: __________ | Repetitions: __________

2. Pose Name: _________________________________ | Duration: __________ | Repetitions: __________

3. Pose Name: _________________________________ | Duration: __________ | Repetitions: __________

4. Pose Name: _________________________________ | Duration: __________ | Repetitions: __________

5. Pose Name: _________________________________ | Duration: __________ | Repetitions: __________

6. Pose Name: _________________________________ | Duration: __________ | Repetitions: __________

Somatic Focus Areas:

☐ Neck and Shoulders | ☐ Spine and Back | ☐ Hips and Pelvis

☐ Legs and Feet | ☐ Arms and Hands | ☐ Full Body Integration

Breathing Techniques Used:

Technique: ____ | Duration: _____________

Post-Session Reflection

Physical Observations:

Flexibility improvements: ____

Strength improvements: ____

Stress level changes: ____

Emotional Observations:

Mood after practice: ____

Emotional shifts: ____

Nutrition:

Breakfast: _______________________________________/Calorie: _________

Snacks: ____/Calorie: _________

Lunch: ____/Calorie: ________

Dinner: ____/ Calorie: _______

Additional Notes:

____

____

____

____

____

Progress Tracking

Weight Tracking:

Weight today: _______________ | Goal weight: ____

Flexibility Tracking:

Forward bend reach: _______________________________ | Goal: _______________________

Strength Tracking:

Hold time for core poses: _____________________________ | Goal: _____________________

Stress Management:

Stress level (1-10): _____________________________ | Goal: _____________________

Overall Well-being (1-10): ____

Goals for Next Session

____
____
____
____
____
____
____
____
____
____
____
____
____

Somatic Yoga Practice Journal

Name: ____/ Date: ____________________

Morning Reflection:

Mood upon waking: _______________________Physical sensations: ___________________

Intentions for today's practice: ____

Yoga Session

Time of Practice: _______________________

Poses Practiced:

1. Pose Name: _______________________ | Duration: _________ | Repetitions: _________

2. Pose Name: _______________________ | Duration: _________ | Repetitions: _________

3. Pose Name: _______________________ | Duration: _________ | Repetitions: _________

4. Pose Name: _______________________ | Duration: _________ | Repetitions: _________

5. Pose Name: _______________________ | Duration: _________ | Repetitions: _________

6. Pose Name: _______________________ | Duration: _________ | Repetitions: _________

Somatic Focus Areas:

☐ Neck and Shoulders | ☐ Spine and Back | ☐ Hips and Pelvis

☐ Legs and Feet | ☐ Arms and Hands | ☐ Full Body Integration

Breathing Techniques Used:

Technique: _______________________________________ | Duration: ___________

Post-Session Reflection

Physical Observations:

Flexibility improvements: ____

Strength improvements: ____

Stress level changes: ____

Emotional Observations:

Mood after practice: ____

Emotional shifts: ____

Nutrition:

Breakfast: _______________________________________/Calorie: _________

Snacks: _______________________________________/Calorie: _________

Lunch: _______________________________________/Calorie: _________

Dinner: _______________________________________/ Calorie: _________

Additional Notes:

____

____

____

____

____

Progress Tracking

Weight Tracking:

Weight today: _________________ | Goal weight: ____

Flexibility Tracking:

Forward bend reach: _________________________________ | Goal: _________________________________

Strength Tracking:

Hold time for core poses: _______________________________ | Goal: _____________________________

Stress Management:

Stress level (1-10): _________________________________ | Goal: _________________________________

Overall Well-being (1-10): ____

Goals for Next Session

____

____

____

____

____

____

____

____

____

____

____

____

Somatic Yoga Practice Journal

Name: ____/ Date: ____________________

Morning Reflection:

Mood upon waking: ________________________________Physical sensations: ____________________

Intentions for today's practice: ____

Yoga Session

Time of Practice: _______________________________

Poses Practiced:

1. Pose Name: ______________________________ | Duration: _________ | Repetitions: _________

2. Pose Name: ______________________________ | Duration: _________ | Repetitions: _________

3. Pose Name: ______________________________ | Duration: _________ | Repetitions: _________

4. Pose Name: ______________________________ | Duration: _________ | Repetitions: _________

5. Pose Name: ______________________________ | Duration: _________ | Repetitions: _________

6. Pose Name: ______________________________ | Duration: _________ | Repetitions: _________

Somatic Focus Areas:

☐ Neck and Shoulders | ☐ Spine and Back | ☐ Hips and Pelvis

☐ Legs and Feet | ☐ Arms and Hands | ☐ Full Body Integration

Breathing Techniques Used:

Technique: ____ | Duration: ____________

Post-Session Reflection

Physical Observations:

Flexibility improvements: ____

Strength improvements: ____

Stress level changes: ____

Emotional Observations:

Mood after practice: ____

Emotional shifts: ____

Nutrition:

Breakfast: _______________________________________/Calorie: _________

Snacks: _______________________________________/Calorie: _________

Lunch: _______________________________________/Calorie: _______

Dinner: _______________________________________/ Calorie: ______

Additional Notes:

____

____

____

____

____

Weight Tracking:

Weight today: _______________ | Goal weight: ____

Flexibility Tracking:

Forward bend reach: _________________________________ | Goal: _______________________________

Strength Tracking:

Hold time for core poses: _________________________________ | Goal: _______________________

Stress Management:

Stress level (1-10): _________________________________ | Goal: _______________________

Overall Well-being (1-10): ____

Goals for Next Session

____
____
____
____
____
____
____
____
____
____
____
____
____

Somatic Yoga Practice Journal

Name: ____ / **Date:** ___________________

Morning Reflection:

Mood upon waking: _______________________Physical sensations: _______________________

Intentions for today's practice: ____

Yoga Session

Time of Practice: _______________________

Poses Practiced:

1. Pose Name: _______________________ | Duration: _________ | Repetitions: _________

2. Pose Name: _______________________ | Duration: _________ | Repetitions: _________

3. Pose Name: _______________________ | Duration: _________ | Repetitions: _________

4. Pose Name: _______________________ | Duration: _________ | Repetitions: _________

5. Pose Name: _______________________ | Duration: _________ | Repetitions: _________

6. Pose Name: _______________________ | Duration: _________ | Repetitions: _________

Somatic Focus Areas:

☐ Neck and Shoulders | ☐ Spine and Back | ☐ Hips and Pelvis

☐ Legs and Feet | ☐ Arms and Hands | ☐ Full Body Integration

Breathing Techniques Used:

Technique: ____ | Duration: ___________

Physical Observations:

Flexibility improvements: ____

Strength improvements: ____

Stress level changes: ____

Emotional Observations:

Mood after practice: ____

Emotional shifts: ____

Nutrition:

Breakfast: ____/Calorie: ________

Snacks: ____/Calorie: ________

Lunch: ____/Calorie: ________

Dinner: ____/ Calorie: ______

Additional Notes:

____

____

____

____

____

Progress Tracking

Weight Tracking:

Weight today: _______________ | Goal weight: ____

Flexibility Tracking:

Forward bend reach: _______________________________ | Goal: _______________________________

Strength Tracking:

Hold time for core poses: _______________________________ | Goal: _______________________

Stress Management:

Stress level (1-10): _______________________________ | Goal: _______________________________

Overall Well-being (1-10): ____

Goals for Next Session

____

____

____

____

____

____

____

____

____

____

____

Somatic Yoga Practice Journal

Name: ____/ **Date:** _____________________

Morning Reflection:

Mood upon waking: _____________________________Physical sensations: _____________________

Intentions for today's practice: ____

Yoga Session

Time of Practice: _______________________________

Poses Practiced:

1. Pose Name: _________________________________ | Duration: _________ | Repetitions: _________

2. Pose Name: _________________________________ | Duration: _________ | Repetitions: _________

3. Pose Name: _________________________________ | Duration: _________ | Repetitions: _________

4. Pose Name: _________________________________ | Duration: _________ | Repetitions: _________

5. Pose Name: _________________________________ | Duration: _________ | Repetitions: _________

6. Pose Name: _________________________________ | Duration: _________ | Repetitions: _________

Somatic Focus Areas:

☐ Neck and Shoulders | ☐ Spine and Back | ☐ Hips and Pelvis

☐ Legs and Feet | ☐ Arms and Hands | ☐ Full Body Integration

Breathing Techniques Used:

Technique: ____ | Duration: _____________

Physical Observations:

Flexibility improvements: ____

Strength improvements: ____

Stress level changes: ____

Emotional Observations:

Mood after practice: ____

Emotional shifts: ____

Nutrition:

Breakfast: _______________________________________/Calorie: _________

Snacks: _______________________________________/Calorie: _________

Lunch: _______________________________________/Calorie: _______

Dinner: _______________________________________/ Calorie: ______

Additional Notes:

____

____

____

____

____

Weight Tracking:

Weight today: _______________ | Goal weight: ____

Flexibility Tracking:

Forward bend reach: _________________________________ | Goal: ______________________________

Strength Tracking:

Hold time for core poses: _______________________________ | Goal: ______________________________

Stress Management:

Stress level (1-10): _______________________________ | Goal: ______________________________

Overall Well-being (1-10): ____

Goals for Next Session

____
____
____
____
____
____
____
____
____
____
____
____
____

Somatic Yoga Practice Journal

Name: _______________________________________/ **Date:** _____________________

Morning Reflection:

Mood upon waking: _______________________________Physical sensations: _______________________

Intentions for today's practice: ____

Yoga Session

Time of Practice: _______________________________

Poses Practiced:

1. Pose Name: _________________________________ | Duration: ___________ | Repetitions: __________

2. Pose Name: _________________________________ | Duration: ___________ | Repetitions: __________

3. Pose Name: _________________________________ | Duration: ___________ | Repetitions: __________

4. Pose Name: _________________________________ | Duration: ___________ | Repetitions: __________

5. Pose Name: _________________________________ | Duration: ___________ | Repetitions: __________

6. Pose Name: _________________________________ | Duration: ___________ | Repetitions: __________

Somatic Focus Areas:

☐ Neck and Shoulders | ☐ Spine and Back | ☐ Hips and Pelvis

☐ Legs and Feet | ☐ Arms and Hands | ☐ Full Body Integration

Breathing Techniques Used:

Technique: ____ | Duration: _____________

Physical Observations:

Flexibility improvements: ____

Strength improvements: ____

Stress level changes: ____

Emotional Observations:

Mood after practice: ____

Emotional shifts: ____

Nutrition:

Breakfast: _______________________________________/Calorie: _________

Snacks: _______________________________________/Calorie: _________

Lunch: _______________________________________/Calorie: _________

Dinner: _______________________________________/ Calorie: _______

Additional Notes:

____

____

____

____

____

Progress Tracking

Weight Tracking:

Weight today: ________________ | Goal weight: ____

Flexibility Tracking:

Forward bend reach: _________________________________ | Goal: _______________________

Strength Tracking:

Hold time for core poses: _______________________________ | Goal: ___________________

Stress Management:

Stress level (1-10): ___________________________________ | Goal: ____________________

Overall Well-being (1-10): ____

Goals for Next Session

____

____

____

____

____

____

____

____

____

____

____

____

Somatic Yoga Practice Journal

Name: ____ / **Date:** ___________________________

Morning Reflection:

Mood upon waking: ______________________________Physical sensations: ______________________________

Intentions for today's practice: ____

Yoga Session

Time of Practice: _________________________________

Poses Practiced:

1. Pose Name: ______________________________ | Duration: __________ | Repetitions: __________

2. Pose Name: ______________________________ | Duration: __________ | Repetitions: __________

3. Pose Name: ______________________________ | Duration: __________ | Repetitions: __________

4. Pose Name: ______________________________ | Duration: __________ | Repetitions: __________

5. Pose Name: ______________________________ | Duration: __________ | Repetitions: __________

6. Pose Name: ______________________________ | Duration: __________ | Repetitions: __________

Somatic Focus Areas:

☐ Neck and Shoulders | ☐ Spine and Back | ☐ Hips and Pelvis

☐ Legs and Feet | ☐ Arms and Hands | ☐ Full Body Integration

Breathing Techniques Used:

Technique: ____ | Duration: ______________

Post-Session Reflection

Physical Observations:

Flexibility improvements: ____

Strength improvements: ____

Stress level changes: ____

Emotional Observations:

Mood after practice: ____

Emotional shifts: ____

Nutrition:

Breakfast: _______________________________________/Calorie: _________

Snacks: _______________________________________/Calorie: _________

Lunch: _______________________________________/Calorie: _______

Dinner: _______________________________________/ Calorie: ______

Additional Notes:

____

____

____

____

____

Progress Tracking

Weight Tracking:

Weight today: _______________ | Goal weight: ____

Flexibility Tracking:

Forward bend reach: _________________________________ | Goal: _______________________________

Strength Tracking:

Hold time for core poses: _____________________________ | Goal: ____________________________

Stress Management:

Stress level (1-10): __________________________________ | Goal: ____________________________

Overall Well-being (1-10): ____

Goals for Next Session

____
____
____
____
____
____
____
____
____
____
____
____
____
____

Somatic Yoga Practice Journal

Name: ____/ **Date:** ____________________

Morning Reflection:

Mood upon waking: ______________________________Physical sensations: ______________________

Intentions for today's practice: ____

Yoga Session

Time of Practice: _______________________________

Poses Practiced:

1. Pose Name: _________________________________ | Duration: __________ | Repetitions: __________

2. Pose Name: _________________________________ | Duration: __________ | Repetitions: __________

3. Pose Name: _________________________________ | Duration: __________ | Repetitions: __________

4. Pose Name: _________________________________ | Duration: __________ | Repetitions: __________

5. Pose Name: _________________________________ | Duration: __________ | Repetitions: __________

6. Pose Name: _________________________________ | Duration: __________ | Repetitions: __________

Somatic Focus Areas:

☐ Neck and Shoulders | ☐ Spine and Back | ☐ Hips and Pelvis

☐ Legs and Feet | ☐ Arms and Hands | ☐ Full Body Integration

Breathing Techniques Used:

Technique: ____ | Duration: ____________

Post-Session Reflection

Physical Observations:

Flexibility improvements: ____

Strength improvements: ____

Stress level changes: ____

Emotional Observations:

Mood after practice: ____

Emotional shifts: ____

Nutrition:

Breakfast: _______________________________/Calorie: ________

Snacks: _______________________________/Calorie: ________

Lunch: _______________________________/Calorie: ________

Dinner: _______________________________/ Calorie: ________

Additional Notes:

____

____

____

____

____

Progress Tracking

Weight Tracking:

Weight today: ________________ | Goal weight: ____

Flexibility Tracking:

Forward bend reach: ________________________________ | Goal: ____________________________

Strength Tracking:

Hold time for core poses: ______________________________ | Goal: ________________________

Stress Management:

Stress level (1-10): ________________________________ | Goal: ____________________________

Overall Well-being (1-10): ____

Goals for Next Session

____

____

____

____

____

____

____

____

____

____

____

Somatic Yoga Practice Journal

Name: ____ / **Date:** _____________________

Morning Reflection:

Mood upon waking: _______________________________Physical sensations: ___________________________

Intentions for today's practice: ____

Yoga Session

Time of Practice: _______________________________

Poses Practiced:

1. Pose Name: _______________________________ | Duration: _________ | Repetitions: _________

2. Pose Name: _______________________________ | Duration: _________ | Repetitions: _________

3. Pose Name: _______________________________ | Duration: _________ | Repetitions: _________

4. Pose Name: _______________________________ | Duration: _________ | Repetitions: _________

5. Pose Name: _______________________________ | Duration: _________ | Repetitions: _________

6. Pose Name: _______________________________ | Duration: _________ | Repetitions: _________

Somatic Focus Areas:

☐ Neck and Shoulders | ☐ Spine and Back | ☐ Hips and Pelvis

☐ Legs and Feet | ☐ Arms and Hands | ☐ Full Body Integration

Breathing Techniques Used:

Technique: ____ | Duration: _____________

Post-Session Reflection

Physical Observations:

Flexibility improvements: ____

Strength improvements: ____

Stress level changes: ____

Emotional Observations:

Mood after practice: ____

Emotional shifts: ____

Nutrition:

Breakfast: _______________________________________/Calorie: _________

Snacks: _______________________________________/Calorie: _________

Lunch: _______________________________________/Calorie: _______

Dinner: _______________________________________/ Calorie: ______

Additional Notes:

____

____

____

____

____

Progress Tracking

Weight Tracking:

Weight today: _______________ | Goal weight: ____

Flexibility Tracking:

Forward bend reach: _________________________________ | Goal: _________________________

Strength Tracking:

Hold time for core poses: _________________________________ | Goal: _________________________

Stress Management:

Stress level (1-10): _________________________________ | Goal: _________________________

Overall Well-being (1-10): ____

Goals for Next Session

____

Somatic Yoga Practice Journal

Name: ____/ **Date:** _____________________

Morning Reflection:

Mood upon waking: _______________________________Physical sensations: ______________________________

Intentions for today's practice: ____

Yoga Session

Time of Practice: _______________________________

Poses Practiced:

1. Pose Name: _________________________________ | Duration: _____________ | Repetitions: _____________

2. Pose Name: _________________________________ | Duration: _____________ | Repetitions: _____________

3. Pose Name: _________________________________ | Duration: _____________ | Repetitions: _____________

4. Pose Name: _________________________________ | Duration: _____________ | Repetitions: _____________

5. Pose Name: _________________________________ | Duration: _____________ | Repetitions: _____________

6. Pose Name: _________________________________ | Duration: _____________ | Repetitions: _____________

Somatic Focus Areas:

☐ Neck and Shoulders | ☐ Spine and Back | ☐ Hips and Pelvis

☐ Legs and Feet | ☐ Arms and Hands | ☐ Full Body Integration

Breathing Techniques Used:

Technique: ____ | Duration: _____________

Post-Session Reflection

Physical Observations:

Flexibility improvements: ____

Strength improvements: ____

Stress level changes: ____

Emotional Observations:

Mood after practice: ____

Emotional shifts: ____

Nutrition:

Breakfast: _______________________________________/Calorie: _________

Snacks: _______________________________________/Calorie: _________

Lunch: _______________________________________/Calorie: _______

Dinner: _______________________________________/ Calorie: ______

Additional Notes:

____

____

____

____

____

Progress Tracking

Weight Tracking:

Weight today: ________________ | Goal weight: ____

Flexibility Tracking:

Forward bend reach: _________________________________ | Goal: _______________________

Strength Tracking:

Hold time for core poses: _____________________________ | Goal: _____________________

Stress Management:

Stress level (1-10): _________________________________ | Goal: _____________________

Overall Well-being (1-10): ____

Goals for Next Session

____
____
____
____
____
____
____
____
____
____
____

Somatic Yoga Practice Journal

Name: ____/ **Date:** _____________________

Morning Reflection:

Mood upon waking: _______________________________Physical sensations: _____________________

Intentions for today's practice: ____

Yoga Session

Time of Practice: _________________________________

Poses Practiced:

1. Pose Name: _______________________________ | Duration: _________ | Repetitions: _________

2. Pose Name: _______________________________ | Duration: _________ | Repetitions: _________

3. Pose Name: _______________________________ | Duration: _________ | Repetitions: _________

4. Pose Name: _______________________________ | Duration: _________ | Repetitions: _________

5. Pose Name: _______________________________ | Duration: _________ | Repetitions: _________

6. Pose Name: _______________________________ | Duration: _________ | Repetitions: _________

Somatic Focus Areas:

☐ Neck and Shoulders | ☐ Spine and Back | ☐ Hips and Pelvis

☐ Legs and Feet | ☐ Arms and Hands | ☐ Full Body Integration

Breathing Techniques Used:

Technique: ____ | Duration: ____________

Post-Session Reflection

Physical Observations:

Flexibility improvements: ____

Strength improvements: ____

Stress level changes: ____

Emotional Observations:

Mood after practice: ____

Emotional shifts: ____

Nutrition:

Breakfast: ____/Calorie: _________

Snacks: ____/Calorie: _________

Lunch: ____/Calorie: ________

Dinner: ____/ Calorie: _______

Additional Notes:

____

____

____

____

____

Progress Tracking

Weight Tracking:

Weight today: _______________ | Goal weight: ____

Flexibility Tracking:

Forward bend reach: _________________________________ | Goal: _______________________

Strength Tracking:

Hold time for core poses: ______________________________ | Goal: _____________________

Stress Management:

Stress level (1-10): _________________________________ | Goal: _______________________

Overall Well-being (1-10): ____

Goals for Next Session

____

____

____

____

____

____

____

____

____

____

____

____

Somatic Yoga Practice Journal

Name: ____ / Date: _______________________

Morning Reflection:

Mood upon waking: _______________________________Physical sensations: _______________________

Intentions for today's practice: ____

Yoga Session

Time of Practice: _______________________________

Poses Practiced:

1. Pose Name: _______________________________ | Duration: _________ | Repetitions: _________

2. Pose Name: _______________________________ | Duration: _________ | Repetitions: _________

3. Pose Name: _______________________________ | Duration: _________ | Repetitions: _________

4. Pose Name: _______________________________ | Duration: _________ | Repetitions: _________

5. Pose Name: _______________________________ | Duration: _________ | Repetitions: _________

6. Pose Name: _______________________________ | Duration: _________ | Repetitions: _________

Somatic Focus Areas:

☐ Neck and Shoulders | ☐ Spine and Back | ☐ Hips and Pelvis

☐ Legs and Feet | ☐ Arms and Hands | ☐ Full Body Integration

Breathing Techniques Used:

Technique: ____ | Duration: _____________

Post-Session Reflection

Physical Observations:

Flexibility improvements: ____

Strength improvements: ____

Stress level changes: ____

Emotional Observations:

Mood after practice: ____

Emotional shifts: ____

Nutrition:

Breakfast: _______________________________________/Calorie: _________

Snacks: _______________________________________/Calorie: _________

Lunch: _______________________________________/Calorie: _________

Dinner: _______________________________________/ Calorie: _______

Additional Notes:

____

____

____

____

____

Progress Tracking

Weight Tracking:

Weight today: _______________ | Goal weight: ____

Flexibility Tracking:

Forward bend reach: _________________________________ | Goal: _______________________

Strength Tracking:

Hold time for core poses: _____________________________ | Goal: ____________________

Stress Management:

Stress level (1-10): _________________________________ | Goal: _____________________

Overall Well-being (1-10): ____

Goals for Next Session

____

____

____

____

____

____

____

____

____

____

____

Somatic Yoga Practice Journal

Name: ____/ **Date:** ____________________

Morning Reflection:

Mood upon waking: _______________________Physical sensations: ____________________

Intentions for today's practice: ____

Yoga Session

Time of Practice: _______________________

Poses Practiced:

1. Pose Name: _______________________ | Duration: _________ | Repetitions: _________

2. Pose Name: _______________________ | Duration: _________ | Repetitions: _________

3. Pose Name: _______________________ | Duration: _________ | Repetitions: _________

4. Pose Name: _______________________ | Duration: _________ | Repetitions: _________

5. Pose Name: _______________________ | Duration: _________ | Repetitions: _________

6. Pose Name: _______________________ | Duration: _________ | Repetitions: _________

Somatic Focus Areas:

☐ Neck and Shoulders | ☐ Spine and Back | ☐ Hips and Pelvis

☐ Legs and Feet | ☐ Arms and Hands | ☐ Full Body Integration

Breathing Techniques Used:

Technique: _______________________________________ | Duration: ___________

Physical Observations:

Flexibility improvements: ______________________________________

Strength improvements: ______________________________________

Stress level changes: ______________________________________

Emotional Observations:

Mood after practice: ______________________________________

Emotional shifts: ______________________________________

Nutrition:

Breakfast: ______________________________/Calorie: ________

Snacks: ______________________________/Calorie: ________

Lunch: ______________________________/Calorie: ________

Dinner: ______________________________/ Calorie: ________

Additional Notes:

____

____

____

____

____

Progress Tracking

Weight Tracking:

Weight today: _______________ | Goal weight: ____

Flexibility Tracking:

Forward bend reach: _________________________________ | Goal: _______________________________

Strength Tracking:

Hold time for core poses: _________________________________ | Goal: _______________________

Stress Management:

Stress level (1-10): _________________________________ | Goal: _______________________

Overall Well-being (1-10): ____

Goals for Next Session

____
____
____
____
____
____
____
____
____
____
____
____

Somatic Yoga Practice Journal

Name: ____/ **Date:** _____________________

Morning Reflection:

Mood upon waking: ______________________________Physical sensations: ____________________________

Intentions for today's practice: ____

Yoga Session

Time of Practice: _______________________________

Poses Practiced:

1. Pose Name: _______________________________ | Duration: __________ | Repetitions: __________

2. Pose Name: _______________________________ | Duration: __________ | Repetitions: __________

3. Pose Name: _______________________________ | Duration: __________ | Repetitions: __________

4. Pose Name: _______________________________ | Duration: __________ | Repetitions: __________

5. Pose Name: _______________________________ | Duration: __________ | Repetitions: __________

6. Pose Name: _______________________________ | Duration: __________ | Repetitions: __________

Somatic Focus Areas:

☐ Neck and Shoulders | ☐ Spine and Back | ☐ Hips and Pelvis

☐ Legs and Feet | ☐ Arms and Hands | ☐ Full Body Integration

Breathing Techniques Used:

Technique: ____ | Duration: ______________

Post-Session Reflection

Physical Observations:

Flexibility improvements: ____

Strength improvements: ____

Stress level changes: ____

Emotional Observations:

Mood after practice: ____

Emotional shifts: ____

Nutrition:

Breakfast: _____________________________________/Calorie: _________

Snacks: ____/Calorie: _________

Lunch: ____/Calorie: _________

Dinner: ____/ Calorie: _______

Additional Notes:

____

____

____

____

____

Progress Tracking

Weight Tracking:

Weight today: _______________ | Goal weight: ____

Flexibility Tracking:

Forward bend reach: _________________________________ | Goal: _____________________________

Strength Tracking:

Hold time for core poses: _______________________________ | Goal: _________________________

Stress Management:

Stress level (1-10): _________________________________ | Goal: ___________________________

Overall Well-being (1-10): ____

Goals for Next Session

____
____
____
____
____
____
____
____
____
____
____
____

Somatic Yoga Practice Journal

Name: ____/ Date: ____________________

Morning Reflection:

Mood upon waking: _______________________Physical sensations: ____________________

Intentions for today's practice: ____

Yoga Session

Time of Practice: _______________________

Poses Practiced:

1. Pose Name: _________________________ | Duration: _________ | Repetitions: _________

2. Pose Name: _________________________ | Duration: _________ | Repetitions: _________

3. Pose Name: _________________________ | Duration: _________ | Repetitions: _________

4. Pose Name: _________________________ | Duration: _________ | Repetitions: _________

5. Pose Name: _________________________ | Duration: _________ | Repetitions: _________

6. Pose Name: _________________________ | Duration: _________ | Repetitions: _________

Somatic Focus Areas:

☐ Neck and Shoulders | ☐ Spine and Back | ☐ Hips and Pelvis

☐ Legs and Feet | ☐ Arms and Hands | ☐ Full Body Integration

Breathing Techniques Used:

Technique: ____ | Duration: ____________

Post-Session Reflection

Physical Observations:

Flexibility improvements: _______________________________________

Strength improvements: _______________________________________

Stress level changes: _______________________________________

Emotional Observations:

Mood after practice: _______________________________________

Emotional shifts: _______________________________________

Nutrition:

Breakfast: _______________________________/Calorie: _______

Snacks: _______________________________/Calorie: _______

Lunch: _______________________________/Calorie: _______

Dinner: _______________________________/ Calorie: _______

Additional Notes:

____

____

____

____

____

Progress Tracking

Weight Tracking:

Weight today: _______________ | Goal weight: ____

Flexibility Tracking:

Forward bend reach: _____________________________ | Goal: _______________________

Strength Tracking:

Hold time for core poses: _____________________________ | Goal: _______________________

Stress Management:

Stress level (1-10): _____________________________ | Goal: _______________________

Overall Well-being (1-10): ____

Goals for Next Session

____
____
____
____
____
____
____
____
____
____
____
____

Somatic Yoga Practice Journal

Name: _______________________________________ / **Date:** _______________________

Morning Reflection:

Mood upon waking: _______________________________Physical sensations: _______________________

Intentions for today's practice: ____

Yoga Session

Time of Practice: _________________________________

Poses Practiced:

1. Pose Name: _________________________________ | Duration: __________ | Repetitions: __________

2. Pose Name: _________________________________ | Duration: __________ | Repetitions: __________

3. Pose Name: _________________________________ | Duration: __________ | Repetitions: __________

4. Pose Name: _________________________________ | Duration: __________ | Repetitions: __________

5. Pose Name: _________________________________ | Duration: __________ | Repetitions: __________

6. Pose Name: _________________________________ | Duration: __________ | Repetitions: __________

Somatic Focus Areas:

☐ Neck and Shoulders | ☐ Spine and Back | ☐ Hips and Pelvis

☐ Legs and Feet | ☐ Arms and Hands | ☐ Full Body Integration

Breathing Techniques Used:

Technique: ____ | Duration: ____________

Post-Session Reflection

Physical Observations:

Flexibility improvements: ____

Strength improvements: ____

Stress level changes: ____

Emotional Observations:

Mood after practice: ____

Emotional shifts: ____

Nutrition:

Breakfast: ____________________________________/Calorie: _________

Snacks: _______________________________________/Calorie: _________

Lunch: ____/Calorie: _________

Dinner: _______________________________________/ Calorie: _______

Additional Notes:

____

____

____

____

____

Progress Tracking

Weight Tracking:

Weight today: _________________ | Goal weight: ____

Flexibility Tracking:

Forward bend reach: _________________________________ | Goal: _________________________________

Strength Tracking:

Hold time for core poses: _________________________ | Goal: _________________________________

Stress Management:

Stress level (1-10): _________________________________ | Goal: _________________________________

Overall Well-being (1-10): ____

Goals for Next Session

____
____
____
____
____
____
____
____
____
____
____
____

Somatic Yoga Practice Journal

Name: ____/ Date: ____________________

Morning Reflection:

Mood upon waking: _______________________Physical sensations: ___________________

Intentions for today's practice: ____

Yoga Session

Time of Practice: _______________________

Poses Practiced:

1. Pose Name: _______________________ | Duration: _________ | Repetitions: _________

2. Pose Name: _______________________ | Duration: _________ | Repetitions: _________

3. Pose Name: _______________________ | Duration: _________ | Repetitions: _________

4. Pose Name: _______________________ | Duration: _________ | Repetitions: _________

5. Pose Name: _______________________ | Duration: _________ | Repetitions: _________

6. Pose Name: _______________________ | Duration: _________ | Repetitions: _________

Somatic Focus Areas:

☐ Neck and Shoulders | ☐ Spine and Back | ☐ Hips and Pelvis

☐ Legs and Feet | ☐ Arms and Hands | ☐ Full Body Integration

Breathing Techniques Used:

Technique: _______________________________________ | Duration: ____________

Post-Session Reflection

Physical Observations:

Flexibility improvements: ____

Strength improvements: ____

Stress level changes: ____

Emotional Observations:

Mood after practice: ____

Emotional shifts: ____

Nutrition:

Breakfast: ____/Calorie: ________

Snacks: ____/Calorie: ________

Lunch: ____/Calorie: ________

Dinner: ____/ Calorie: ______

Additional Notes:

____

____

____

____

____

Progress Tracking

Weight Tracking:

Weight today: _______________ | Goal weight: ____

Flexibility Tracking:

Forward bend reach: _______________________________ | Goal: _______________________

Strength Tracking:

Hold time for core poses: _______________________ | Goal: _______________________

Stress Management:

Stress level (1-10): _______________________________ | Goal: _______________________

Overall Well-being (1-10): ____

Goals for Next Session

____
____
____
____
____
____
____
____
____
____
____
____
____

Somatic Yoga Practice Journal

Name: _______________________________________/ Date: ___________________

Morning Reflection:

Mood upon waking: _______________________Physical sensations: ___________________________

Intentions for today's practice: ____

Yoga Session

Time of Practice: _______________________________

Poses Practiced:

1. Pose Name: _____________________________ | Duration: _________ | Repetitions: _________

2. Pose Name: _____________________________ | Duration: _________ | Repetitions: _________

3. Pose Name: _____________________________ | Duration: _________ | Repetitions: _________

4. Pose Name: _____________________________ | Duration: _________ | Repetitions: _________

5. Pose Name: _____________________________ | Duration: _________ | Repetitions: _________

6. Pose Name: _____________________________ | Duration: _________ | Repetitions: _________

Somatic Focus Areas:

☐ Neck and Shoulders | ☐ Spine and Back | ☐ Hips and Pelvis

☐ Legs and Feet | ☐ Arms and Hands | ☐ Full Body Integration

Breathing Techniques Used:

Technique: ____ | Duration: ___________

Post-Session Reflection

Physical Observations:

Flexibility improvements: ____

Strength improvements: ____

Stress level changes: ____

Emotional Observations:

Mood after practice: ____

Emotional shifts: ____

Nutrition:

Breakfast: ____/Calorie: _________

Snacks: ____/Calorie: _________

Lunch: ____/Calorie: _________

Dinner: ____/ Calorie: _______

Additional Notes:

____

____

____

____

____

Progress Tracking

Weight Tracking:

Weight today: _______________ | Goal weight: ____

Flexibility Tracking:

Forward bend reach: _________________________________ | Goal: _______________________

Strength Tracking:

Hold time for core poses: _______________________________ | Goal: ___________________

Stress Management:

Stress level (1-10): _________________________________ | Goal: _______________________

Overall Well-being (1-10): ____

Goals for Next Session

____
____
____
____
____
____
____
____
____
____
____
____
____

Somatic Yoga Practice Journal

Name: ____ / **Date:** ___________________

Morning Reflection:

Mood upon waking: _______________________________Physical sensations: ___________________________

Intentions for today's practice: ____

Yoga Session

Time of Practice: _______________________________

Poses Practiced:

1. Pose Name: _______________________________ | Duration: __________ | Repetitions: __________

2. Pose Name: _______________________________ | Duration: __________ | Repetitions: __________

3. Pose Name: _______________________________ | Duration: __________ | Repetitions: __________

4. Pose Name: _______________________________ | Duration: __________ | Repetitions: __________

5. Pose Name: _______________________________ | Duration: __________ | Repetitions: __________

6. Pose Name: _______________________________ | Duration: __________ | Repetitions: __________

Somatic Focus Areas:

☐ Neck and Shoulders | ☐ Spine and Back | ☐ Hips and Pelvis

☐ Legs and Feet | ☐ Arms and Hands | ☐ Full Body Integration

Breathing Techniques Used:

Technique: ____ | Duration: ____________

Post-Session Reflection

Physical Observations:

Flexibility improvements: ____

Strength improvements: ____

Stress level changes: ____

Emotional Observations:

Mood after practice: ____

Emotional shifts: ____

Nutrition:

Breakfast: _______________________________________/Calorie: _________

Snacks: _______________________________________/Calorie: _________

Lunch: _______________________________________/Calorie: _________

Dinner: _______________________________________/ Calorie: ______

Additional Notes:

____

____

____

____

____

Progress Tracking

Weight Tracking:

Weight today: _______________ | Goal weight: ____

Flexibility Tracking:

Forward bend reach: _________________________________ | Goal: _______________________________

Strength Tracking:

Hold time for core poses: _______________________________ | Goal: _______________________________

Stress Management:

Stress level (1-10): _________________________________ | Goal: _______________________________

Overall Well-being (1-10): ____

Goals for Next Session

____
____
____
____
____
____
____
____
____
____
____
____
____
____

Somatic Yoga Practice Journal

Name: _______________________________________ **/ Date:** _______________________

Morning Reflection:

Mood upon waking: _______________________________Physical sensations: _______________________

Intentions for today's practice: ____

Yoga Session

Time of Practice: _______________________________

Poses Practiced:

1. Pose Name: _______________________________ | Duration: __________ | Repetitions: __________

2. Pose Name: _______________________________ | Duration: __________ | Repetitions: __________

3. Pose Name: _______________________________ | Duration: __________ | Repetitions: __________

4. Pose Name: _______________________________ | Duration: __________ | Repetitions: __________

5. Pose Name: _______________________________ | Duration: __________ | Repetitions: __________

6. Pose Name: _______________________________ | Duration: __________ | Repetitions: __________

Somatic Focus Areas:

☐ Neck and Shoulders | ☐ Spine and Back | ☐ Hips and Pelvis

☐ Legs and Feet | ☐ Arms and Hands | ☐ Full Body Integration

Breathing Techniques Used:

Technique: ____ | Duration: _____________

Post-Session Reflection

Physical Observations:

Flexibility improvements: ____

Strength improvements: ____

Stress level changes: ____

Emotional Observations:

Mood after practice: ____

Emotional shifts: ____

Nutrition:

Breakfast: _______________________________________/Calorie: ________

Snacks: _______________________________________/Calorie: ________

Lunch: _______________________________________/Calorie: ________

Dinner: _______________________________________/ Calorie: ______

Additional Notes:

____

____

____

____

____

Progress Tracking

Weight Tracking:

Weight today: _______________ | Goal weight: ____

Flexibility Tracking:

Forward bend reach: _________________________________ | Goal: _____________________________

Strength Tracking:

Hold time for core poses: _____________________________ | Goal: _____________________________

Stress Management:

Stress level (1-10): _________________________________ | Goal: _____________________________

Overall Well-being (1-10): ____

Goals for Next Session

____

____

____

____

____

____

____

____

____

____

____

____

Somatic Yoga Practice Journal

Name: _______________________________________/ **Date:** ___________________________

Morning Reflection:

Mood upon waking: _______________________________Physical sensations: _____________________________

Intentions for today's practice: ____

Yoga Session

Time of Practice: _______________________________

Poses Practiced:

1. Pose Name: _________________________________ | Duration: __________ | Repetitions: __________

2. Pose Name: _________________________________ | Duration: __________ | Repetitions: __________

3. Pose Name: _________________________________ | Duration: __________ | Repetitions: __________

4. Pose Name: _________________________________ | Duration: __________ | Repetitions: __________

5. Pose Name: _________________________________ | Duration: __________ | Repetitions: __________

6. Pose Name: _________________________________ | Duration: __________ | Repetitions: __________

Somatic Focus Areas:

☐ Neck and Shoulders | ☐ Spine and Back | ☐ Hips and Pelvis

☐ Legs and Feet | ☐ Arms and Hands | ☐ Full Body Integration

Breathing Techniques Used:

Technique: ____ | Duration: _____________

Post-Session Reflection

Physical Observations:

Flexibility improvements: ____

Strength improvements: ____

Stress level changes: ____

Emotional Observations:

Mood after practice: ____

Emotional shifts: ____

Nutrition:

Breakfast: ____________________________/Calorie: ________

Snacks: ____________________________/Calorie: ________

Lunch: ____________________________/Calorie: ________

Dinner: ____________________________/ Calorie: ______

Additional Notes:

____

____

____

____

____

Progress Tracking

Weight Tracking:

Weight today: _______________ | Goal weight: ____________________________________

Flexibility Tracking:

Forward bend reach: _________________________________ | Goal: _______________________

Strength Tracking:

Hold time for core poses: _______________________________ | Goal: ____________________

Stress Management:

Stress level (1-10): _________________________________ | Goal: ______________________

Overall Well-being (1-10): ____

Goals for Next Session

____

____

____

____

____

____

____

____

____

____

____

____

Somatic Yoga Practice Journal

Name: ______________________________________/ **Date:** ____________________

Morning Reflection:

Mood upon waking: _______________________________Physical sensations: ____________________________

Intentions for today's practice: ____

Yoga Session

Time of Practice: ___________________________

Poses Practiced:

1. Pose Name: _______________________________ | Duration: __________ | Repetitions: __________

2. Pose Name: _______________________________ | Duration: __________ | Repetitions: __________

3. Pose Name: _______________________________ | Duration: __________ | Repetitions: __________

4. Pose Name: _______________________________ | Duration: __________ | Repetitions: __________

5. Pose Name: _______________________________ | Duration: __________ | Repetitions: __________

6. Pose Name: _______________________________ | Duration: __________ | Repetitions: __________

Somatic Focus Areas:

☐ Neck and Shoulders | ☐ Spine and Back | ☐ Hips and Pelvis

☐ Legs and Feet | ☐ Arms and Hands | ☐ Full Body Integration

Breathing Techniques Used:

Technique: ____ | Duration: ____________

Post-Session Reflection

Physical Observations:

Flexibility improvements: ____

Strength improvements: ____

Stress level changes: ____

Emotional Observations:

Mood after practice: ____

Emotional shifts: ____

Nutrition:

Breakfast: ____/Calorie: ________

Snacks: ____/Calorie: ________

Lunch: ____/Calorie: ________

Dinner: ____/ Calorie: ________

Additional Notes:

____

____

____

____

____

Progress Tracking

Weight Tracking:

Weight today: _______________ | Goal weight: ____

Flexibility Tracking:

Forward bend reach: _________________________________ | Goal: _______________________

Strength Tracking:

Hold time for core poses: _____________________________ | Goal: _____________________

Stress Management:

Stress level (1-10): _________________________________ | Goal: _____________________

Overall Well-being (1-10): ____

Goals for Next Session

____
____
____
____
____
____
____
____
____
____
____
____

Somatic Yoga Practice Journal

Name: ____/ **Date:** ____________________

Morning Reflection:

Mood upon waking: ______________________________Physical sensations: ____________________________

Intentions for today's practice: ____

Yoga Session

Time of Practice: ______________________________

Poses Practiced:

1. Pose Name: _________________________________ | Duration: __________ | Repetitions: __________

2. Pose Name: _________________________________ | Duration: __________ | Repetitions: __________

3. Pose Name: _________________________________ | Duration: __________ | Repetitions: __________

4. Pose Name: _________________________________ | Duration: __________ | Repetitions: __________

5. Pose Name: _________________________________ | Duration: __________ | Repetitions: __________

6. Pose Name: _________________________________ | Duration: __________ | Repetitions: __________

Somatic Focus Areas:

☐ Neck and Shoulders | ☐ Spine and Back | ☐ Hips and Pelvis

☐ Legs and Feet | ☐ Arms and Hands | ☐ Full Body Integration

Breathing Techniques Used:

Technique: ____ | Duration: ____________

Post-Session Reflection

Physical Observations:

Flexibility improvements: ____

Strength improvements: ____

Stress level changes: ____

Emotional Observations:

Mood after practice: ____

Emotional shifts: ____

Nutrition:

Breakfast: _______________________________________/Calorie: _________

Snacks: _______________________________________/Calorie: _________

Lunch: _______________________________________/Calorie: _________

Dinner: _______________________________________/ Calorie: _______

Additional Notes:

____

____

____

____

____

Progress Tracking

Weight Tracking:

Weight today: ________________ | Goal weight: ____

Flexibility Tracking:

Forward bend reach: _________________________________ | Goal: _______________________

Strength Tracking:

Hold time for core poses: ______________________________ | Goal: _____________________

Stress Management:

Stress level (1-10): _________________________________ | Goal: _______________________

Overall Well-being (1-10): ____

Goals for Next Session

____
____
____
____
____
____
____
____
____
____
____
____

Somatic Yoga Practice Journal

Name: ____/ **Date:** ____________________

Morning Reflection:

Mood upon waking: ___________________________Physical sensations: ______________________

Intentions for today's practice: ____

Yoga Session

Time of Practice: _______________________________

Poses Practiced:

1. Pose Name: ______________________________ | Duration: __________ | Repetitions: __________

2. Pose Name: ______________________________ | Duration: __________ | Repetitions: __________

3. Pose Name: ______________________________ | Duration: __________ | Repetitions: __________

4. Pose Name: ______________________________ | Duration: __________ | Repetitions: __________

5. Pose Name: ______________________________ | Duration: __________ | Repetitions: __________

6. Pose Name: ______________________________ | Duration: __________ | Repetitions: __________

Somatic Focus Areas:

☐ Neck and Shoulders | ☐ Spine and Back | ☐ Hips and Pelvis

☐ Legs and Feet | ☐ Arms and Hands | ☐ Full Body Integration

Breathing Techniques Used:

Technique: ____ | Duration: ____________

Post-Session Reflection

Physical Observations:

Flexibility improvements: ____

Strength improvements: ____

Stress level changes: ____

Emotional Observations:

Mood after practice: ____

Emotional shifts: ____

Nutrition:

Breakfast: ____/Calorie: _________

Snacks: ____/Calorie: _________

Lunch: ____/Calorie: _________

Dinner: ____/ Calorie: _______

Additional Notes:

____

____

____

____

____

Progress Tracking

Weight Tracking:

Weight today: _______________ | Goal weight: ___________________________________

Flexibility Tracking:

Forward bend reach: _______________________________ | Goal: _______________________

Strength Tracking:

Hold time for core poses: ____________________________ | Goal: ____________________

Stress Management:

Stress level (1-10): ______________________________ | Goal: ______________________

Overall Well-being (1-10): ____

Goals for Next Session

____

____

____

____

____

____

____

____

____

____

____

____

Somatic Yoga Practice Journal

Name: _______________________________________/ **Date:** __________________

Morning Reflection:

Mood upon waking: _______________________Physical sensations: __________________

Intentions for today's practice: ____

Yoga Session

Time of Practice: _______________________

Poses Practiced:

1. Pose Name: _______________________ | Duration: _________ | Repetitions: _________

2. Pose Name: _______________________ | Duration: _________ | Repetitions: _________

3. Pose Name: _______________________ | Duration: _________ | Repetitions: _________

4. Pose Name: _______________________ | Duration: _________ | Repetitions: _________

5. Pose Name: _______________________ | Duration: _________ | Repetitions: _________

6. Pose Name: _______________________ | Duration: _________ | Repetitions: _________

Somatic Focus Areas:

☐ Neck and Shoulders | ☐ Spine and Back | ☐ Hips and Pelvis

☐ Legs and Feet | ☐ Arms and Hands | ☐ Full Body Integration

Breathing Techniques Used:

Technique: _______________________________________ | Duration: ____________

Post-Session Reflection

Physical Observations:

Flexibility improvements: ____

Strength improvements: ____

Stress level changes: ____

Emotional Observations:

Mood after practice: ____

Emotional shifts: ____

Nutrition:

Breakfast: _______________________________________/Calorie: _________

Snacks: _______________________________________/Calorie: _________

Lunch: _______________________________________/Calorie: _________

Dinner: _______________________________________/ Calorie: _______

Additional Notes:

____

____

____

____

____

Progress Tracking

Weight Tracking:

Weight today: _______________ | Goal weight: ____

Flexibility Tracking:

Forward bend reach: _______________________________ | Goal: ______________________________

Strength Tracking:

Hold time for core poses: _______________________________ | Goal: ______________________

Stress Management:

Stress level (1-10): _______________________________ | Goal: ______________________________

Overall Well-being (1-10): ____

Goals for Next Session

____
____
____
____
____
____
____
____
____
____
____
____

Somatic Yoga Practice Journal

Name: ____ / **Date:** ____________________

Morning Reflection:

Mood upon waking: ________________________________Physical sensations: ______________________________

Intentions for today's practice: ____

Yoga Session

Time of Practice: ________________________________

Poses Practiced:

1. Pose Name: _______________________________ | Duration: __________ | Repetitions: __________

2. Pose Name: _______________________________ | Duration: __________ | Repetitions: __________

3. Pose Name: _______________________________ | Duration: __________ | Repetitions: __________

4. Pose Name: _______________________________ | Duration: __________ | Repetitions: __________

5. Pose Name: _______________________________ | Duration: __________ | Repetitions: __________

6. Pose Name: _______________________________ | Duration: __________ | Repetitions: __________

Somatic Focus Areas:

☐ Neck and Shoulders | ☐ Spine and Back | ☐ Hips and Pelvis

☐ Legs and Feet | ☐ Arms and Hands | ☐ Full Body Integration

Breathing Techniques Used:

Technique: ____ | Duration: ____________

Physical Observations:

Flexibility improvements: ____

Strength improvements: ____

Stress level changes: ____

Emotional Observations:

Mood after practice: ____

Emotional shifts: ____

Nutrition:

Breakfast: _________________________________/Calorie: _______

Snacks: _________________________________/Calorie: _______

Lunch: _________________________________/Calorie: _______

Dinner: _________________________________/ Calorie: ______

Additional Notes:

____

____

____

____

____

Progress Tracking

Weight Tracking:

Weight today: _______________ | Goal weight: ____

Flexibility Tracking:

Forward bend reach: _________________________________ | Goal: _______________________

Strength Tracking:

Hold time for core poses: _____________________________ | Goal: _____________________

Stress Management:

Stress level (1-10): _________________________________ | Goal: _______________________

Overall Well-being (1-10): ____

Goals for Next Session

____
____
____
____
____
____
____
____
____
____
____
____

Somatic Yoga Practice Journal

Name: ____/ Date: _______________________

Morning Reflection:

Mood upon waking: _______________________________Physical sensations: _______________________

Intentions for today's practice: ____

Yoga Session

Time of Practice: _______________________________

Poses Practiced:

1. Pose Name: _______________________________ | Duration: _________ | Repetitions: _________

2. Pose Name: _______________________________ | Duration: _________ | Repetitions: _________

3. Pose Name: _______________________________ | Duration: _________ | Repetitions: _________

4. Pose Name: _______________________________ | Duration: _________ | Repetitions: _________

5. Pose Name: _______________________________ | Duration: _________ | Repetitions: _________

6. Pose Name: _______________________________ | Duration: _________ | Repetitions: _________

Somatic Focus Areas:

☐ Neck and Shoulders | ☐ Spine and Back | ☐ Hips and Pelvis

☐ Legs and Feet | ☐ Arms and Hands | ☐ Full Body Integration

Breathing Techniques Used:

Technique: ____ | Duration: _____________

Post-Session Reflection

Physical Observations:

Flexibility improvements: ____

Strength improvements: ____

Stress level changes: ____

Emotional Observations:

Mood after practice: ____

Emotional shifts: ____

Nutrition:

Breakfast: _______________________________________/Calorie: _________

Snacks: _______________________________________/Calorie: _________

Lunch: _______________________________________/Calorie: _________

Dinner: _______________________________________/ Calorie: _______

Additional Notes:

____

____

____

____

____

Weight Tracking:

Weight today: _______________ | Goal weight: ____

Flexibility Tracking:

Forward bend reach: _________________________________ | Goal: _______________________________

Strength Tracking:

Hold time for core poses: _______________________________ | Goal: ___________________________

Stress Management:

Stress level (1-10): _________________________________ | Goal: ______________________________

Overall Well-being (1-10): ____

Goals for Next Session

____
____
____
____
____
____
____
____
____
____
____
____

30 Day Somatic Yoga Routing

A 30-day workout plan focusing on Somatic Yoga practice. This plan is designed to gently introduce you to the practice, gradually building your strength and flexibility. Remember to start each session with a warm-up and end with a cool-down to prevent injuries.

Day	Focus Area	Activity	Duration
1	Full Body	Gentle Somatic Yoga Flow	20 mins
2	Relaxation	Somatic Breathing Exercises	15 mins
3	Neck and Shoulders	Somatic Shoulder Roll and Neck Release	15 mins
4	Back	Somatic Back Release	20 mins
5	Core	Somatic Core Activation	20 mins
6	Hips and Hamstrings	Somatic Hip Opener and Hamstring Stretch	20 mins

7	Rest and Restore	Somatic Relaxation and Breath work	15 mins
8	Full Body	Dynamic Somatic Movement	25 mins
9	Flexibility	Somatic Stretching	20 mins
10	Balance	Standing Somatic Yoga Poses	20 mins
11	Neck and Shoulders	Somatic Neck and Shoulder Release	15 mins
12	Back	Somatic Spinal Twist	20 mins
13	Lower Body	Somatic Leg and Hip Series	20 mins
14	Upper Body	Somatic Arm and Shoulder Series	20 mins
15	Hips and Hamstrings	Somatic Hip Flexor Release	20 mins

16	Full Body	Somatic Body Scan and Release	25 mins
17	Rest and Restore	Somatic Deep Relaxation & Mindful Meditation	15 mins
18	Neck and Shoulders	Somatic Shoulder Opener	15 mins
19	Back	Somatic Back-bend	20 mins
20	Core	Somatic Core Stability	25 mins
21	Balance	Standing Somatic Yoga Poses	20 min
22	Full Body	Somatic Total Body Integration	25 mins
23	Side Body Stretch	Extended Side Angle Sequence	10 mins
24	Relaxation	Somatic Breathing Exercises	15 mins

25	Hips and Hamstrings	Somatic Hamstring Release | Somatic Hip Flexibility	20 mins
26	Neck and Shoulders	Somatic Neck and Shoulder Mobility	15 mins
27	Back	Somatic Back Strength | Somatic Spinal Release	25 mins
28	Core	Somatic Core Connection | Somatic Core Release	25 mins
29	Rest and Restore	Mindful Meditation | Somatic Breath work and Meditation	30 mins
30	Integration	Full Somatic Yoga Sequence	60 mins

Your 30-Day Nutritional Plan

Day	Meal	Breakfast	Lunch	Dinner	Snacks	Water
1	Balanced	Greek yogurt with berries and honey	Quinoa salad with vegetables and grilled chicken	Baked salmon with sweet potato and steamed broccoli	Apple slices with almond butter	8 glasses
2	Protein-rich	Scrambled eggs with spinach and whole grain toast	Lentil soup with whole grain bread	Grilled turkey breast with quinoa and roasted veggies	Greek yogurt with granola	8 glasses
3	Fiber and Protein	Overnight oats with chia seeds, almond milk, and fruit	Chickpea salad with mixed greens	Baked chicken with brown rice and asparagus	Mixed nuts and dried fruit	8 glasses
4	Antioxidant-rich	Smoothie with spinach, berries, banana, and protein powder	Turkey and avocado wrap with whole grain tortilla	Baked cod with quinoa and roasted Brussels sprouts	Carrot sticks with hummus	8 glasses
5	Energy-boosting	Whole grain pancakes with Greek yogurt and fruit	Grilled vegetable quinoa bowl	Stir-fried tofu with vegetables and brown rice	Rice cakes with peanut butter	8 glasses
6	Hydration-focused	Chia seed pudding with coconut milk and berries	Green salad with grilled chicken	Baked sweet potato with black beans and avocado	Greek yogurt with honey	8 glasses
7	Rest and Digest	Banana almond smoothie	Lentil and vegetable stew	Grilled salmon with quinoa and steamed broccoli	Apple slices with almond butter	8 glasses
8	Balanced	Oatmeal with nuts and dried fruit	Turkey and vegetable stir-fry	Baked chicken with quinoa and roasted vegetables	Greek yogurt with granola	8 glasses
9	Protein-rich	Scrambled tofu with spinach and whole grain toast	Lentil salad with mixed greens	Grilled turkey breast with quinoa and roasted veggies	Mixed nuts and dried fruit	8 glasses

Day	Meal	Breakfast	Lunch	Dinner	Snacks	Water
10	Fiber and Protein	Smoothie bowl with protein powder, fruit, and nuts	Chickpea and vegetable curry	Baked cod with brown rice and roasted Brussels sprouts	Carrot sticks with hummus	8 glasses
11	Antioxidant-rich	Acai bowl with granola and berries	Turkey and avocado salad	Baked chicken with quinoa and steamed asparagus	Rice cakes with peanut butter	8 glasses
12	Energy-boosting	Whole grain toast with avocado and poached eggs	Grilled vegetable and quinoa wrap	Stir-fried tofu with vegetables and brown rice	Apple slices with almond butter	8 glasses
13	Hydration-focused	Smoothie with coconut water, spinach, and berries	Green salad with grilled chicken	Baked sweet potato with black beans and avocado	Greek yogurt with honey	8 glasses
14	Rest and Digest	Chia seed pudding with almond milk and berries	Lentil and vegetable stew	Grilled salmon with quinoa and steamed broccoli	Mixed nuts and dried fruit	8 glasses
15	Balanced	Greek yogurt with granola and honey	Quinoa and black bean salad	Baked chicken with sweet potato and steamed broccoli	Carrot sticks with hummus	8 glasses
16	Protein-rich	Scrambled eggs with spinach and whole grain toast	Lentil soup with whole grain bread	Grilled turkey breast with quinoa and roasted veggies	Rice cakes with peanut butter	8 glasses
17	Fiber and Protein	Overnight oats with chia seeds, almond milk, and fruit	Chickpea salad with mixed greens	Baked cod with quinoa and roasted Brussels sprouts	Apple slices with almond butter	8 glasses
18	Antioxidant-rich	Smoothie with spinach, berries, banana, and protein powder	Turkey and avocado wrap with whole grain tortilla	Baked chicken with brown rice and asparagus	Greek yogurt with granola	8 glasses
19	Energy-	Whole grain pancakes	Grilled vegetable quinoa	Stir-fried tofu with	Mixed nuts and	8 glasses

Day	Meal	Breakfast	Lunch	Dinner	Snacks	Water
	boosting	with Greek yogurt and fruit	bowl	vegetables and brown rice	dried fruit	
20	Hydration-focused	Chia seed pudding with coconut milk and berries	Green salad with grilled chicken	Baked sweet potato with black beans and avocado	Rice cakes with peanut butter	8 glasses
21	Rest and Digest	Banana almond smoothie	Lentil and vegetable stew	Grilled salmon with quinoa and steamed broccoli	Apple slices with almond butter	8 glasses
22	Balanced	Oatmeal with nuts and dried fruit	Turkey and vegetable stir-fry	Baked chicken with quinoa and roasted vegetables	Greek yogurt with granola	8 glasses
23	Protein-rich	Scrambled tofu with spinach and whole grain toast	Lentil salad with mixed greens	Grilled turkey breast with quinoa and roasted veggies	Mixed nuts and dried fruit	8 glasses
24	Fiber and Protein	Smoothie bowl with protein powder, fruit, and nuts	Chickpea and vegetable curry	Baked cod with brown rice and roasted Brussels sprouts	Carrot sticks with hummus	8 glasses
25	Antioxidant-rich	Acai bowl with granola and berries	Turkey and avocado salad	Baked chicken with quinoa and steamed asparagus	Rice cakes with peanut butter	8 glasses
26	Energy-boosting	Whole grain toast with avocado and poached eggs	Grilled vegetable and quinoa wrap	Stir-fried tofu with vegetables and brown rice	Apple slices with almond butter	8 glasses
27	Hydration-focused	Smoothie with coconut water, spinach, and berries	Green salad with grilled chicken	Baked sweet potato with black beans and avocado	Greek yogurt with honey	8 glasses
28	Rest and Digest	Chia seed pudding with almond milk and berries	Lentil and vegetable stew	Grilled salmon with quinoa and steamed	Mixed nuts and dried fruit	8 glasses

Day	Meal	Breakfast	Lunch	Dinner	Snacks	Water
				broccoli		
29	Balanced	Greek yogurt with granola and honey	Quinoa and black bean salad	Baked chicken with sweet potato and steamed broccoli	Carrot sticks with hummus	8 glasses
30	Protein-rich	Scrambled eggs with spinach and whole grain toast	Lentil soup with whole grain bread	Grilled turkey breast with quinoa and roasted veggies	Rice cakes with peanut butter	8 glasses

Conclusion

Somatic Yoga Exercises for Weight Loss offers a holistic approach to achieving and maintaining a healthy weight. Through gentle yet effective somatic yoga practices, this book guides you on a journey of self-discovery, helping you reconnect with your body and mind.

By incorporating mindfulness, breath work, and movement, somatic yoga goes beyond traditional exercise routines. It helps you develop a deeper understanding of your body's needs and signals, empowering you to make conscious choices that support your weight loss goals.

Throughout this book, you've learned how somatic yoga can enhance your metabolism, improve flexibility and mobility, reduce stress, and balance your emotions. These practices are not just about physical exercise; they're about cultivating a positive relationship with yourself and your body.

As you continue your somatic yoga journey, remember that progress is not always linear. Be patient and kind to yourself, and celebrate every small victory along the way. With dedication and perseverance, you'll not only achieve your weight loss goals but also discover a newfound sense of balance, vitality, and well-being.

Wishing You Good Luck